环球卓越
www.geedu.com
（优路教育旗下品牌）

卓越医学考博英语应试教材
ZHUOYUE ENGLISH TEST PREPARATION FOR FATMD

2023

18天攻克 医学考博

英语核心词

主 编：环球卓越医学考博命题研究中心
主 编：梁莉娟 赵牧童

U0385589

机械工业出版社
CHINA MACHINE PRESS

本书作为已有良好市场声誉的卓越医学考博英语应试教材的单本。由全国知名医学博士英语统考培训机构"环球卓越"策划，联手医学博士资深辅导专家，在对近10年真题词频统计的基础上，结合大纲要求，对词频为3以上的单词进行精选、精讲，并针对医学考生时间紧、战线长、记忆压力大等现实情况，将学习任务分解成18天，化整为零，去粗取精，内容精炼。同时本书配套音频朗读，加之口袋大小的设计，携带便捷，考生随时随地可记忆单词。

图书在版编目（CIP）数据

18天攻克医学考博英语核心词／环球卓越医学考博命题研究中心组编；梁莉娟，赵牧童编著. —北京：机械工业出版社，2022.6
　ISBN 978 - 7 - 111 - 70978 - 7

　Ⅰ.①1… 　Ⅱ.①环… ②梁… ③赵… 　Ⅲ.①医学-英语-词汇-博士生入学考试-自学参考资料 Ⅳ.①R

中国版本图书馆 CIP 数据核字（2022）第 099109 号

机械工业出版社（北京市百万庄大街22号　邮政编码100037）
策划编辑：孙铁军　　　　　责任编辑：孙铁军
责任校对：苏筛琴　　　　　责任印制：张　博
中教科（保定）印刷股份有限公司印刷

2022年7月第1版第1次印刷
105mm×148mm·4.125 印张·157 千字
标准书号：ISBN 978 - 7 - 111 - 70978 - 7
定价：32.80 元

电话服务　　　　　　　　　网络服务
客服电话：010 - 88361066　机 工 官 网：www.cmpbook.com
　　　　　010 - 88379833　机 工 官 博：weibo.com/cmp1952
　　　　　010 - 68326294　金 书 网：www.golden-book.com
封底无防伪标均为盗版　机工教育服务网：www.cmpedu.com

丛书序

　　这是一套由全国知名医学博士英语统考培训机构"环球卓越"（优路教育旗下品牌）策划，联手医学博士英语资深辅导专家，为众多志在考取医学博士的考生量身定制的应试辅导用书。国家医学考试中心于2019年底修订了考试大纲，对全国医学博士外语统一考试的题型及各部分分值进行了局部调整。新大纲仍然设置了听力对话、听力短文、词语用法、完形填空、阅读理解和书面表达6种题型，但调整了具体命题形式，其中听力部分变化最大。"15个短对话＋1个长对话＋2个短文"的经典组合成为历史，从2020年开始，"5个短对话＋5个小短文"的搭配将在很长一段时间内成为考生要面对的题型。考试时间为3个小时（含播放录音及收发卷时间）。

　　考纲的变化并未改变对考生能力的考查方向，因此为了帮助广大考生在较短的时间内系统备考，在听、说、读、写4个方面得到强化训练，全面提高英语应用和交际能力，顺利通过考试，本套"卓越医学考博英语应试教材"仍然是广大考生朋友们很好的选择。本丛书于紧密结合最近几年卫生部组织的医学博士英语统一考试命题情况，针对最新考试大纲进行了修订，并针对新题型编写了大量针对性练习。为应对新题型的变化，2021年丛书在《全国医学博士英语统考词汇巧战通关》《全国医学博士英语统考综合应试教程》《全国医学博士英语统考实战演练》《医学考博阅读理解高分全解》和《医学考博听力、完形、写作高分全解》5个传统分册的基础上，特意增加了《医学考博英语听力28天训练计划》。为了应对新冠疫情带来的考试时间的不确定性，本丛书在2023版增加了《18天攻克医学考博英语核心词》的小分册，帮助考生们在短时间内掌握重点词汇。传统分册从基础到综合再到真题实战，从写作、完形等细分模块到全套仿真试题，对分值较大的阅读理解单立分册进行详解精练，让考生在有限的时间里快速准确地把握每一个进度，28天听力分册则根据听力训练的规律和要点，按天设置训练内容，有助于考生在考前做好全面细致的准备，顺利攻克考试难关，获得高分。

本丛书的特点如下：

一、紧贴考试，实用性强

策划编写本丛书的作者常年在教学一线授课，从基础英语到医博考前辅导，积累了大量的应试辅导实战经验。丛书内容是他们多年辅导经验的提炼和结晶，实用性非常强，专为医学考博考生定制，是目前市面上较全面、系统的医学考博英语应试教材。

二、紧扣大纲，直击真题

本丛书紧扣最新大纲，体例设置与大纲保持一致；各部分考点紧密结合最新历年真题，还原真实考场环境，命题思路分析透彻，重点突出，讲解精确；各部分内容严格控制在大纲规定的范围之内，让考生准确把握考试的重点、难点及命题趋势。

三、内容精练，讲练结合

传统分册《全国医学博士英语统考词汇巧战通关》《全国医学博士英语统考综合应试教程》和《全国医学博士英语统考实战演练》简单精练，通过突破词汇基础关、学习各个题型应试方法以及在高质量实战中历练，考生可在有限的时间内进行全面复习，把握重点，比系统地完成考前准备。模块分册《医学考博阅读理解高分全解》和《医学考博听力、完形、写作高分全解》则是根据考生的具体情况，分模块予以详解，提升基础，总结技巧，各个击破。听力专项《医学考博英语听力 28 天训练计划》则专练听力，循序渐进，按天分配学习任务，力争高分。核心词汇专项《18 天攻克医学考博英语核心词》在使用词频软件完整统计近十年的全套真题的基础上，将该统计结果和大纲词汇进行比较，最后确定出记忆任务的内容和安排。按天设置，不断重复。

四、超值服务，锦上添花

本丛书附带赠送精品服务，由优路教育为每位购书读者提供专业的服务和强大的技术支持。具体为：

1.《医学考博英语听力28天训练计划》附赠内容：优路教育"2023年医学考博（统考）《英语听力28天训练计划》图书赠课英语（20节）"网络视频课程。使用方法：刮卡书籍封面的兑换码，扫描书籍封面二维码关注【优路医学考试】微信公众账号后，点击【兑换课程】—【点击这里兑换课程】的链接，输入兑换码，输入姓名手机号，将自动跳转至您的课程页，开始观看课程。后续看课路径：关注【优路医学考试】服务号，在底部菜单栏【我要学习】—【我的课程】查看课程。（可通过扫描本页下方二维码，关注后兑换课程）

2.《18天攻克医学考博英语核心词》附赠内容：优路教育"2023年医学考博（统考）《18天攻克医学考博英语核心词》图书赠课英语（20节）"网络视频课程。使用方法：刮卡书籍封面的兑换码，扫描书籍封面二维码关注【优路医学考试】微信公众账号后，点击【兑换课程】—【点击这里兑换课程】的链接，输入兑换码，输入姓名手机号，将自动跳转至您的课程页，开始观看课程。后续看课路径：关注【优路医学考试】服务号，在底部菜单栏【我要学习】—【我的课程】

查看课程。（可通过扫描本页下方二维码，关注后兑换课程）

3.《全国医学博士英语统考实战演练》附赠内容：优路教育"2023年 医学考博（统考）《实战演练》图书赠课英语（10节）"网络视 频课程。使用方法：刮卡书籍封面的兑换码，扫描书籍封面二维码关注【优路医学考试】微信公众账号后，点击【兑换课程】-【点击这里兑换课程】的链接，输入兑换码，输入姓名手机号，将自动跳转至您的课程页，开始观看课程。后续看课路径：关注【优路医学考试】服务号，在底部菜单栏【我要学习】-【我的课程】查看课程。（可通过扫描本页下方二维码，关注后兑换课程）

4.《全国医学博士英语统考综合应试教程》附赠内容：优路教育"2023年医学考博（统考）《综合应试教程》图书赠课英语（10节）"网络视频课程。使用方法：刮卡书籍封面的兑换码，扫描书籍封面二维码关注【优路医学考试】微信公众账号后，点击【兑换课程】-【点击这里兑换课程】的链接，输入姓名手机号，将自动跳转至您的课程页，开始观看课程。后续看课路径：关注【优路医学考试】服务号，在底部菜单栏【我要学习】-【我的课程】查看课程。（可通过扫描本页下方二维码，关注后兑换课程）

5.《全国医学博士英语统考综词汇巧战通关》附赠内容：优路教育"2023年医学考博（统考）《词汇巧战通关》图书赠课【学习卡】英语（10节）"网络视频课

程。使用方法：刮卡书籍封面的兑换码，扫描书籍封面二维码关注【优路医学考试】微信公众账号后，点击【兑换课程】－【点击这里兑换课程】的链接，输入兑换码，输入姓名手机号，将自动跳转至您的课程页，开始观看课程。后续看课路径：关注【优路医学考试】服务号，在底部菜单栏【我要学习】－【我的课程】查看课程。（可通过扫描本页下方二维码，关注后兑换课程）

6.《医学考博听力、完形、写作高分全解》附赠内容：优路教育"2023 年医学考博（统考）《听力、完形、写作高分全解》图书赠课【学习卡】英语（10节）"网络视频课程。使用方法：刮卡书籍封面的兑换码，扫描书籍封面二维码关注【优路医学考试】微信公众账号后，点击【兑换课程】－【点击这里兑换课程】的链接，输入兑换码，输入姓名手机号，将自动跳转至您的课程页，开始观看课程。后续看课路径：关注【优路医学考试】服务号，在底部菜单栏【我要学习】－【我的课程】查看课程。（可通过扫描本页下方二维码，关注后兑换课程）

7.《医学考博阅读理解高分全解》附赠内容：优路教育"2023 年医学考博（统考）《阅读理解高分全解》图书赠课【学习卡】英语（8节）"网络视频课程。使用方法：刮卡书籍封面的兑换码，扫描书籍封面二维码关注【优路医学考试】微信公众账号后，点击【兑换课程】－【点击这里兑换课程】的链接，输入兑换码，输入姓名手机号，将自动跳转至您的课程页，开始观看课程。后续看课路径：关注【优路医学考试】服务号，在底部菜单栏【我要学习】－【我的课程】查看课程。（可通过扫描本页下方二维码，关注后兑换课程）

优路教育技术支持及服务热线 400－8835－981，可以帮您解决兑换及观看课程中的技术问题。您也可以登录优路教育网站 www.youlu.com，在"医学博士英语"栏目下获取更多的学习资料和资讯。

扫码关注后兑换课程

编　者

2022 年 6 月于北京

前　言

　　医学博士入学英语考试的词汇复习是个大难题。"词汇词汇，必须要背"，道理都懂，可考生总在不甘心地四处探寻：背什么？怎么背？作为一个研究英语考试多年的一线英语老师来讲，我着实也无法说出更多天花乱坠的奇妙方法，无法装出手里握着天下无二的记忆妙方的样子。读者们都是准博士了，英语水平先放一边不论，逻辑思维能力和归纳总结水平一定已经炉火纯青了，那么一定能判断，背单词无论是顺序记忆、乱序记忆，抑或词根词缀记忆、谐音记忆，都脱离不了两个字：重复。但重复是要有内涵的。重复两遍5000个词，或许和重复10遍1000个词所用时间相差无几，但结果一定是大相径庭。前者大约能对500个词"有印象"，而后者能将500个词熟稔于心。因此，绝大多数考生都认同且追求把有限的时间用于尽可能少的内容的记忆。

　　这就是编写本书《18天攻克医学考博英语核心词》的基础：浓缩记忆内容，设置重复场景。尽可能地创造"10（遍）×1000（词）"的机会。记忆内容可不能乱减，必须有权威指引和科学基础。研究再三，我们采取了"从真题出发，向大纲进攻"的路径：使用词

目　录

等，本部分采用的是【联想】【搭配】【导学】【例句】的体例，提供不同的记忆路径，以便记忆时能事半功倍。【例句】大多从历年真题中挑选经典句子来讲解词汇，并配有译文。【联想】则是"联想词"和"派生词"，这样做可以让考生开阔视野，举一反三，成串记忆。【搭配】则是该词的特殊用法、习惯搭配等。【导学】重在辨析近义词。

如前所述，附录中放入词频统计的结果全文，大家可自行排序，有参照地复习。同时，将基础词汇的表格版及查询版也放入了附录部分，建议考生们按照筛查的方式唤醒记忆、查漏补缺。如果考生朋友想要更详细的工具书，则可移步《全国医学博士英语统考词汇巧战通关》，那里应有尽有。

本书同时附上词汇朗读音频和讲解视频，不方便用阅读的方式复习的时候，耳朵也是可以随时打开接受英语的"刺激"的，这有助于维持自己复习的状态，将碎片化时间利用到极致。

感谢广大考生和众多老师在编写过程中提供的建议和帮助。由于时间仓促，书中难免有错误及遗漏之处，欢迎批评指正。

编者

2022 年 4 月 12 日

频软件完整统计近十年的全套真题，再将该统计结果和大纲词汇进行比较，最后确定出记忆任务的层次和要求，先搞定真题，再填补和大纲的差距。而对于"重复"的机会，我们则设置成"3周×7-3（休息检测日）"的模式，即18天、每天不到100个单词的单日任务，目的就在于使考生有不断重复的可能性。

从统计结果中不难发现，词频超过10次的，往往是初中词汇（甚至小学词汇），比如排名最前的 the、a、with 等（后附详细统计结果），这些单词的记忆要求层次为"唤醒"，因此我们将接近2000个基础词汇附上词义、词性、固定搭配等置于附录中，并提供测试表格，建议考生打印多份，不断检测、扫描、唤醒，换言之，此部分单词不需要背诵，而是筛查。

按常理，我们应该手握大纲，循序渐进，从头背起。但通过研究真题发现，医学博士入学英语考试的词汇范围，在实际命题中并非严格以大纲为蓝本，考生认为不重要的，不一定是命题人不考的，比如 antidioxide。换言之，四六级的考试经验，未见得完全适用于医博英语考试，毕竟有"医学"这个限定词。基于这种现实情况，我们对词频3~10之间的词汇与大纲进行对照，删掉基础词汇，补进真题词汇，最后形成了我们18天的记忆主体。

18天的记忆任务原则上是按字母排序规划的，但为了减少"顺序记忆"中的心理压力（从 A 到 Z，遥遥无期），我们进行了字母组合，比如 A + Z，B + Q

Day 1

abandon [əˈbændən]　　　　　　*vt.* 放弃，抛弃，离弃

【联想】give up doing sth. / quit doing sth. 放弃做某事

【导学】abandon 后接动名词，如：abandon doing sth. 放弃做某事。

【例句】But even if some disasters meant that the vault was abandoned, the permanently frozen soil would keep the seeds alive.

【译文】但是，即使某些灾难意味着储藏室被遗弃了，永远冰冻的土地也会使种子保持活力。

ability [əˈbiliti]　　　　　　*n.* 能力，智能；才能，才干

【搭配】of great/exceptional ability 能力卓越
of high/low/average ability 能力高/低/一般
to the best of one's ability 尽其所能

【联想】able 能的—unable 不能的
ability 能力—inability 无能
enable 使能够—disable 使无能，使残废

【例题】She soon received a promotion, for her superiors realized that she was a woman of considerable _____.

A. future　　　　B. possibility

1

    C. ability   D. opportunity   C

【译文】她很快得到了提拔，因为她的上级意识到她是一个相当有能力的女人。

abnormal [æbˈnɔːməl]   *a*. 不正常的

【联想】abnormally *ad*. 不正常地

【例句】The so-called Mad Cow Disease is caused by abnormal proteins coming into contact with neurons in the brain.

【译文】所谓"疯牛病"，是异常蛋白质侵入脑神经原引起的。

abolish [əˈbɔliʃ]   *vt*. 废除，取消

【例句】The first step is to abolish the existing system.

【译文】首先要废除现行体制。

abroad [əˈbrɔːd]   *ad*. 国外，海外；传开

【搭配】at home and abroad 国内外

absent [ˈæbsənt]   *a*. 缺席的；缺乏的；漫不经心的

【搭配】be absent from 缺席

【联想】absence *n*. 缺席，缺乏

【例题】So many directors _____, the board meeting had to be put off.

    A. were absent   B. being absent

    C. been absent   D. had been absent   B

【译文】由于太多的董事缺席，董事会议不得不推迟。

absolute ['æbsəlu:t]　　　　　*a*. 绝对的；完全的

【例句】Sometimes we buy a magazine with absolutely no purpose other than to pass time.

【译文】有时我们买杂志是完全没有目的的，仅仅是为了打发时间。

absorb [əb'sɔ:b]　　　　*vt*. 吸收；吸引，使专心

【搭配】be absorbed in 全神贯注于

【联想】absorption *n*. 吸收

【例题】She was so _____ in her job that she didn't hear anybody knocking at the door.

　　A. attracted　　　　B. absorbed

　　C. drawn　　　　　D. concentrated　　　B

【译文】她完全沉浸于工作当中，没有听到任何敲门声。

abuse [ə'bju:s]　　*n*. 滥用；虐待；辱骂；陋习，弊端

　　　　[ə'bju:z]　　　　　　　*vt*. 滥用；虐待；辱骂

【搭配】abuse one's authority 滥用职权

【联想】abuser *n*. 滥用者；abusive *a*. 滥用的

【例句】The abuse of alcohol and drugs is also a common factor.

【译文】酗酒和吸毒是常见的因素。

academic [ˌækəˈdemik]　　　　　*a.* 学院的；学术的

【联想】academia *n.* 学术界；academics *n.* 学术

【例句】The effective work of maintaining discipline is usually performed by students who advise the academic authorities.

【译文】有效地维持纪律通常是由学生来做的，这些学生负责给学校的领导提建议。

accelerate [əkˈseləreit]　　*v.* 加快；加速；（使）加速

【联想】acceleration *n.* 加速，加快

【例句】Growth will accelerate to 2.9 per cent next year.

【译文】明年的增长会加速至2.9%。

acceptance [əkˈseptəns]　　　　*n.* 接受，接纳；承认

【联想】accept *vt.* 接受；acceptable *a.* 可接受的

access [ˈækses]　　*n.* 通路；访问 *vt.* 访问；存取

【搭配】get/gain/have（no）access to（没）有机会或权利得到（接近、进入、使用）

【联想】accessbile *a.* 可接近的

【例题】Finding out about these universities has become easy for anyone with Internet _____.

　　A. entrance　　　　B. admission

　　C. access　　　　　D. entry　　　　　　　C

【译文】对于任何能够上网的人来说，了解这些大学的情况都很容易。

accidental [ˌæksɪˈdentl] *a.* 意外的，偶然（发生）的

【联想】accident *n.* 事故

【例题】While shopping in a department store, I _____ left my purse lying on a counter of handbags.

A. initially   B. fortunately

C. frustratedly   D. accidentally   D

【译文】在商场购物时，我不小心把钱包落在了卖手提包的柜台上。

accomplish [əˈkɒmplɪʃ]   *v.* 完成，实现，达到

【联想】accomplishment *n.* 成就，成绩

【例句】I accomplished two hours' work before dinner.

【译文】我在吃饭前完成了两小时的工作。

accord [əˈkɔːd]   *v.* 给予；允许；使一致

【搭配】according to 按照，根据；据……所说，按……所载

【联想】accordingly *ad.* 依照；由此，于是；相应地

【例句】His opinion accorded with mine.

【译文】他的意见与我的一致。

account [əˈkaunt] 　　　　　*n.* 账，账户；说明，叙述
　　　　　　　　　　　　　　　　　vi. 解释

【搭配】account for 解释；on account of 因为，由于；
on no account 决不；on all accounts 无论如
何；take into account 考虑，重视

【例题】I am afraid that you'll have to _____ the
deterioration of the condition.
A. account for　　　B. call for
C. look for　　　　　D. make for　　　　　Ａ

【译文】恐怕你要对环境恶化做出解释。

accumulate [əˈkjuːmjəleɪt] 　　　*v.* 积累；积聚；
　　　　　　　　　　　（数量）逐渐增加；（数额）逐渐增长

【例句】By investing wisely she accumulated a fortune.

【译文】她投资精明，积累了一笔财富。

accurate [ˈækjurit] 　　　　　*a.* 正确的，精确的

【联想】accuracy *n.* 精确，精准

【例句】Although technically accurate, that is an impersonal assessment.

【译文】虽然从技术上说是精确的，但这是一个不讲人
情的评估。

ache [eik]
vi. 疼痛；隐痛
n. （身体某部位的）疼痛

【例句】Muscular aches and pains can be soothed by a relaxing massage.

【译文】放松按摩可以缓解肌肉疼痛。

achievement [ə'tʃi:vmənt]
n. 完成，达到；成就，成绩

【联想】achieve vt. 达到，取得

【例题】His greatest _____ is to make all the players into a united team.

    A. fulfillment   B. achievement

    C. establishment   D. accomplishment   B

【译文】他最大的成就在于使得所有的队员团结在一起。

acid ['æsid]
n. 酸 a. 酸的

【联想】acidify vt. 酸化

acknowledge [ək'nɔlidʒ]
vt. 承认；感谢；告知收到（信件等）

【联想】acknowledgement n. 承认，感谢

【例句】I acknowledge the truth of his statement.

【译文】我承认他说的是事实。

acquire [ə'kwaiə]   *vt.* 取得，获得；学到

【联想】acquisition *n.* 获得，得到

【例句】Most adults find it extremely difficult to acquire even a basic knowledge, particularly in a short time.

【译文】多数成人发现，即使学会一种基本知识也是非常困难的，尤其是在很短的时间内。

activity [æk'tiviti]   *n.* 活动；活力；行动

activate ['æktiveit]   *vt.* 使活动起来，使开始

【例句】Research discovered that plants infected with a virus give off a gas that activates disease resistance in neighboring plants.

【译文】研究发现，感染了病毒的植物会释放出一种气体，来激活周围植物的疾病抵抗能力。

【导学】近义词：stimulate, initiate, arouse, actuate

adapt [ə'dæpt]   *vt.* 使适应；改编

【搭配】adapt oneself to 使自己适应或习惯于某事

adapt...to 使……适应

【联想】adaptive *a.* 适应的

adaptation *n.* 改编，适应

【例题】In spite of the wide range of reading material

specially written or _____ for language learning purposes, there is yet no comprehensive systematic program for reading skills.

A. adapted   B. acknowledged

C. assembled   D. appointed   A

【译文】虽然有大量的为了语言学习而编写或改编的阅读材料，但是在阅读技巧方面仍然没有全面系统的方案。

addict [əˈdikt]   *vt.* 使成瘾，热衷于

【例句】Many people mistakenly believe the term drug refers only to some sort of medicine or an illegal chemical taken by addicts.

【译文】很多人错误地认为"药物"这个词仅仅指某种药品或是吸毒成瘾者服用的违禁化学品。

addicted [əˈdiktid]   *a.* 对……上瘾的，入迷的

【搭配】be addicted to 对……上瘾，入迷

【联想】addiction *n.* 上瘾，入迷

addition [əˈdiʃən]   *n.* 加，加法；附加部分，增加（物）

【搭配】in addition 另外；in addition to 除……之外

【联想】additional *a.* 附加的，另外的

adequate [ˈædikwit]　　　　　　　*a.* 足够的，充分的

【例句】You are bound to have nights where you don't get an adequate amount of sleep.

【译文】你一定会经历睡眠不足的夜晚的。

adjust [əˈdʒʌst]　　　　　　*v.* 调整，调节；校准
　　　　　　　　　　　　　　vt. (to) 适应于

【搭配】adjust... to 使……适应于

【联想】adjustment *n.* 调整，调节

【例题】As a teacher you have to _____ your methods to suit the needs of slower children.

　　　　A. adopt　　　　B. adjust

　　　　C. adapt　　　　D. acquire　　　　B

【译文】作为教师，你应该调整你的方法去适应反应速度慢的孩子的需求。

Day 2

administer [əd'ministə]　　*vt.* 管理，经营；行政机关

【联想】 administration *n.* 管理

【例句】 In the 3rd International Mathematics and Science Study, 13-year-olds from Singapore achieved the best scores in standardized tests of maths and science that were administered to 287,896 students from 41 countries.

【译文】 在第三届国际数学与科学研究中，来自新加坡的13岁年龄组在数学和科学标准化考试中获得最好成绩，参加该项测试的共有来自41个国家的287896名学生。

admission [əd'miʃən]　　　　　*n.* 允许进入，承认

admonish [əd'mɒniʃ]

　　　　　v. 责备；告诫；警告；力劝；忠告

【例句】 They admonished me for taking risks with my health.

【译文】 他们责备我不应拿自己的健康冒险。

adopt [ə'dɒpt]　　　　*vt.* 收养；采用，采纳；通过

【搭配】 the adopted children 收养的孩子

11

【联想】adoption *n.* 采纳；收养

【例句】Since pollution control measures tend to be money consuming, many industries hesitate to adopt them.

【译文】因为污染控制措施会增加开销，所以很多行业在采取这些措施时都很犹豫。

adult [ə'dʌlt, 'ædʌlt]   *n.* 成人 *a.* 成年的，成熟的

【联想】adulthood *n.* 成年人

【例句】Given that we can not turn the clock back, adults can still do plenty to help the next generation cope.

【译文】虽然我们不能让时光倒流，但成年人仍能够做很多事情帮助下一代应对。

advance [əd'vɑːns]   *n.* /*v.* 前进，行进；进步；进展；预付款；勾引；（价格、价值的）上涨，提高

【联想】advanced *a.* 先进的，高级的

advantage [əd'vɑːntidʒ]   *n.* 优点，有利条件；利益，好处

【搭配】take advantage of 乘……之机，利用
be of advantage to 利于

advertise ['ædvətaiz]   *vt.* 做广告

【例题】I shall _____ the loss of my reading-glasses

in the newspaper with a reward for the finder.

A. advertise   B. inform

C. announce   D. publish   A

【译文】我要在报纸上登一则挂失广告，并对送回我的老花镜的拾到者给予回报。

advisable [əd'vaizəbl]   *a.* 明智的，可取的

【导学】It is advisable that 从句中谓语动词用原形表示虚拟。

advocate ['ædvəkeit]   *vt.* 提倡，鼓吹

        [ædvəkət]   *n.* 提倡者，鼓吹者

【例题】Professor Wu traveled and lectured throughout the country to _____ education and professional skills so that women could enter the public world.

A. prosecute   B. acquire

C. advocate   D. proclaim   C

【译文】吴教授在全国各地巡回演讲，提倡推广对女性的教育及提高其职业技能，以使其走入社会。

aerobic [eə'rəubik]   *a.* 需氧的；好氧的；有氧的；增强心肺功能的

aesthetic [iːsˈθetik]   *a.* 美学的，审美的；
                                          悦目的，雅致的

【例句】The more one is conscious of one's political bias, the more chance one has of acting politically without sacrificing one's aesthetic and intellectual integrity.

【译文】越是意识到自己的政治态度，就越可能按政治行事而同时又不牺牲自己美学和思想上的气节。

affect [əˈfekt] *vt.* 影响，作用；使感动；（疾病）侵袭

【例题】We are interested in the weather because it ＿＿＿＿＿ us so directly—what we wear, what we do, and even how we feel.

　　　　A. affects   B. benefits
　　　　C. guides   D. effects   A

【译文】我们对天气十分感兴趣，因为它直接影响了我们，穿衣、行为，甚至感受。

affection [əˈfekʃən]   *n.* 爱，感情；作用，影响

【搭配】have an affection for sb. 热爱某人

【例句】We know the kiss as a form of expressing affection.

【译文】我们知道亲吻是表达感情的一种方式。

afford [əˈfɔːd]　　　　　　v. 负担得起；提供；买得起；(有时间) 做，能做；承担得起 (后果)；给予

【联想】affordable *a*. 负担得起的，可承受的

【例句】We cannot afford to ignore this warning.

【译文】我们对这个警告绝不能等闲视之。

agency [ˈeidʒənsi]　　　　　　*n*. 代理 (处)，代办 (处)

【例句】The agency developed a campaign that focused on travel experiences such as freedom, escape, relaxation and enjoyment of the great western outdoors.

【译文】这个代理商开展了一项活动，重点关注旅行体验，如在广阔的西部户外旅行的自由、逃离现实的生活、放松和乐趣。

agenda [əˈdʒendə]　　　　　　*n*. 议事日程，记事册

【搭配】put on the agenda 提到议事日程上来

agent [ˈeidʒənt]　　　　　　*n*. 代理人，经办人

【例句】The agent stressed the need to fulfill the order exactly.

【译文】代理人强调要严格按照要求完成订单。

aggravate [ˈæɡrəveit]　　　　　　*vt*. 加重；加剧；使恼火，激怒；使……恶化

aggression [ə'greʃən]　　　　　　　*n*. 侵略，攻击

【联想】aggressive *a*. 侵略的，侵犯的

aid [eid]　　　　　　　　　　　　*vi*. 援助，救援
　　　　　　　　　　　　n. 援助，救护；助手，辅助物

【导学】辨析 aid，assist，help：做动词时，aid 指提供帮助、支援或救助；assist 指"给……帮助"或"支持"，尤指作为隶属或补充；help 的含义较多，表示"给予协助、救助，对……有帮助，（在商店或餐馆中）为……服务，促进，（治疗、药物等）缓解、减轻（疼痛、病症）"；help 为普通词，常可代替 aid、assist。做名词时，aid 指帮助的行为或结果，也指助人者，辅助设备；assist 指助人行为；help 指帮助的行动或实例，或指补救的办法，也指助手、雇工。

ailment ['eilmənt]　　　　　　　*n*. 小病；轻病；小恙

【联想】ail *vi*. 生病

【例句】A surprising number of ailments are caused by unsuspected environmental factors.

【译文】有大量疾病是由不明环境因素造成的。

alarm [ə'lɑːm]　　　　　　　　　*n*. 惊恐；警报；警报器
　　　　　　　　　　　　　vt. 惊动，惊吓；向……报警

alcohol [ˈælkəhɒl]　　　　　　　*n*. 酒精，乙醇

【联想】alcoholic *a*. 含有乙醇的，含有酒精的 *n*. 酒鬼，酗酒者

【例句】Alcohol in excess is still bad for you，but a glass of wine with dinner is probably fine for nonalcoholics.

【译文】过量饮酒对你仍然有害，不过晚餐时喝一杯酒对非嗜酒者恐怕无害。

alert [əˈlɜːt]　　　　　　　*a*. 警觉的 *n*. 警惕
　　　　　　　　　　　　　vt. 使警觉；使意识到

alien [ˈeiljən]　　　　　　　*a*. 外国的，外国人的；陌生的；
　　　　　　　　　　　　　性质不同的，不相容的 *n*. 外国人；外星人

【导学】alien 与 foreign 都含有"外国人"的意思。alien 指住在一个国家，但不是该国公民的人；foreigner 指生于或来自他国者，尤指有不同语言、文化的人。

【例句】We deport aliens who slip across our borders.

【译文】我们把偷渡入境的外国人驱逐出境。

alike [əˈlaik]　　　　　　　*a*. 相同的，相似的

【例题】Exercise seems to benefit the brain power of healthy and sick，young and old _____.

    A. alike   B. alive

    C. together   D. included   A

【译文】 锻炼似乎有益于健康人和病人的智力，无论是
        年轻人还是老年人。

allergey [ˈælədʒi]   *n*. 过敏；变态反应

【联想】 allergic *a*. 过敏的

alleviate [əˈliːvieit]

        vt. 减轻（痛苦等），缓和（情绪）

【例题】 The doctor gave him an injection in order to
        _____ the pain.

    A. alleviate   B. aggregate

    C. abolish   D. allocate   A

【译文】 医生给他注射来减轻疼痛。

alliance [əˈlaiəns]   *n*. 结盟，联盟，联姻

allowance [əˈlauəns]   *n*. 津贴；零用钱

【例题】 His mother gives him a monthly _____ of
        ¥450.

    A. income   B. allowance

    C. wages   D. pay   B

【译文】 他母亲每月给他 450 元的零用钱。

allocate [ˈæləkeit]   *vt*. 分配；拨……（给）；
                              划……（归）

【例句】 More resources are being allocated to the project.

【译文】 正在调拨更多的资源给这个项目。

ally [ə'lai, 'ælai]　　　　　　　*n.* 同盟者；伙伴；同类

alternate ['ɔːltəneit]　　　　　　*v.* 交替，轮流
　　　　　　['ɔːltə:nit]　　　　　　*n.* 代替者；代理人

【导学】 近义词：vary, fluctuate, vacillate, oscillate, waver, seesaw, teeter, shift, sway, totter; rotate, substitute

【例句】 Conversation calls for a willingness to alternate the role of speaker with that of listener, and it calls for occasional "digestive pauses" by both.

【译文】 会话要求说话人与听话人都愿意交换角色，并且需要双方偶尔做出"消化停顿"以理解彼此的意思。

alternative [ɔːl'tə:nətiv]　　　　*a.* 两者选一的
　　　　　　　　　　　　　　　　n. 供选择的东西；取舍

【例题】 There was no _____ but to close the road until February.

　　A. dilemma　　　　B. denying

　　C. alternative　　　D. doubt

C

【译文】除了将道路封闭到 2 月份外，别无选择。

aiter ['ɔ:ltə]　　　　　　　　*vt.* 改变，变更

【导学】辨析 alter, change, convert, modify, shift, transform, vary：alter 指局部、表面的改变，不影响事物的本质或总体结构，如修改衣服的大小等；change 指全部、完全的改变；convert 指由一种形式或用途变为另一种形式或用途；modify 指做小的修改，只能用于改变方法、计划、制度、组织、意思、条款等；shift 指位置或方向的移动、改变；transform 指外貌、性格或性质的彻底改变；vary 多指形式、外表、本质上的繁多而断续的变化或改变，使其多样化。

【例句】With the tools of technology he has altered many physical features of the earth.

【译文】通过一些技术手段，他已经改变了地球的许多物理特征。

amaze [ə'meiz]　　　　　　*vt.* 使惊愕，使惊叹

【导学】辨析 amaze, astonish, surprise, shock：前三个词中，amaze 语气最强，尤其在被认为不可能之事实际上已发生时使用，也可表示"惊奇，惊叹"；astonish 语气稍强，意为"使大吃一惊，使惊愕"，指事情的发生不可

思议而"难以置信"；surprise 是一般用语，指对事出突然或出乎意料而"吃惊，惊奇"；shock 意为"使……震惊，使……惊讶"，指事物的发生出乎意料，使人感到震惊。

amazing [əˈmeiziŋ]　　　　*a.* 令人惊讶的，令人吃惊的

【导学】It's amazing that 从句中的动词用原形或"should＋原形"表示虚拟语气。

【例句】Some people apparently have an amazing ability to come up with the right answer.

【译文】很明显，一些人有惊人的得出正确答案的能力。

Day 3

ambition [æmˈbiʃən]   *n.* 雄心；野心

【联想】ambitious *a.* 野心勃勃的

【例题】These diplomatic principles completely laid bare their _____ for world conquest.

    A. admiration   B. ambition

    C. administration D. orientation   B

【译文】这些外交政策彻底暴露了他们想征服世界的野心。

amid [əˈmid]   *prep.* 在……中，在……当中

amount [əˈmaunt]   *n.* 数据，数额，总数

                                                 vt. (to) 合计，相当于，等同

【搭配】a large amount of（＋不可数名词）大量的

【导学】辨析 number，total，amount：number 和 total 均为及物动词；amount 是不及物动词，须加 to 再跟宾语。

【例句】Getting a proper amount of rest is absolutely essential for increasing your energy.

【译文】适量的休息绝对是增加体能所必需的。

amplify [ˈæmplifai]   *vt.* 放大，增大，扩大

【例句】 By turning this knob to the right you can amplify the sound from the radio.

【译文】 朝右边拧一拧旋钮，你就能放大收音机的声音。

analysis [əˈnælisis]   *n.* 分析，解析

【联想】 analyst *n.* 分析者

analytical *a.* 分析的

analyse *vt.* 分析

【导学】 该词复数形式为 analyses。

【联想】 单复数形式转换：

basis—bases 基础

crisis—crises 危机

thesis—theses 论题

hypothesis—hypotheses 假设

diagnosis—diagnoses 诊断

emphasis—emphases 强调

anatomy [əˈnætəmi] *n.* 解剖学，(动植物的)结构，解剖

ancestor [ˈænsistə]   *n.* 祖宗，祖先

ancient [ˈeinʃənt]   *a.* 古代的，古老的

【例句】 Floods have undermined the foundation of the ancient bridge.

Day 3

【译文】洪水已经侵蚀了古老桥梁的根基。

anesthetic [ˌænəsˈθetik]   *a.* 麻醉的

ankle [ˈæŋkl]   *n.* 踝，踝关节

announcement [əˈnaunsmənt]

                        n. 布告，通告；预告，声明

annoy [əˈnɔi]   *vt.* 使烦恼，使生气，打搅

【例题】At this time of the year, university admission
          offices are _____ with inquiries from
          anxious applicants.
          A. annoyed   B. thrilled
          C. trampled   D. reproached   A

【译文】每逢此时，大学招生办公室都会被考生急切的
          咨询所困扰着。

annual [ˈænjuəl] *a.* 每年的，年度的 *n.* 年刊，年鉴

【联想】daily *n.* 日刊；weekly *n.* 周刊；monthly *n.*
          月刊；quarterly *n.* 季刊；yearly/annual *n.*
          年刊

【例句】The fruit account for more than half the
          country's annual exports, according to a
          recent report.

【译文】根据最新的报告，这种水果的出口量占该国年
          度出口总量的一半以上。

anti- [ˌænti]   *prefix* 反，逆

【联想】 antibody 抗体
          antibiotic 抗生素
          antidepressant 抗抑郁药物
          antioxidant 抗氧化剂
          antiretroviral 抗逆转录病毒

anticipate [æn'tisipeit]   *vt. /vi.* 预料，预计

【例句】 It is anticipated that inflation will stabilize at 3%.
【译文】 据预测，通货膨胀将稳定在3%。

anxiety [æŋg'zaiəti]   *n.* 挂念，焦虑，担心；
                                                        渴望，热望

【联想】 anxious *a.* 焦虑的
【例句】 He was waiting for his brother's return with anxiety.
【译文】 他焦急地等着兄弟归来。

apart [ə'pɑːt]   *ad.* 分离，隔开；相距，相隔

【搭配】 apart from （= besides）除……之外
【联想】 except for 除……之外；in addition to 除……之外；fall apart 土崩瓦解

apology [ə'pɒlədʒi]   *n.* 道歉，歉意

【搭配】 make an apology to sb. for (doing) sth. 为某

25

事向某人道歉

【联想】 apologize *v*. 道歉

appalling [əˈpɔːliŋ]　　*a*. 骇人听闻的，令人震惊的，可怕的

apparent [əˈpærənt]　　　*a*. 明显的；表面的

【搭配】 apparent to 对……是显而易见的

【例句】 It is apparent that the watches that finally arrived have been produced from inferior materials.

【译文】 很明显，最后到货的那批手表是用劣等材料制成的。

appeal [əˈpiːl]　　　　*vi*. (to) 请求，呼吁；吸引；上诉；求助 *n*. 呼吁；吸引力；上诉

【例句】 On the positive side, emotional appeals may respond to a consumer's real concerns.

【译文】 从积极的方面来说，（广告的）情感鼓动也能反映消费者真正的需求。

appearance [əˈpiərəns]　　*n*. 出现，出场，露面；外表，外观

appetite [ˈæpitait]　　　*n*. 食欲，胃口；欲望

【搭配】 have no appetite for work 不想工作

【联想】 have a desire for，have inclination for，long for，be hungry/thirsty for 渴望

appliance [əˈplaiəns]　　　*n*. 用具，设备，器械；装置

【联想】equipment *n*. 设备（不可数）

　　　　instrument *n*. 仪器

　　　　facilities *n*. 设施

apply [əˈplai]　　　　　　　*vi*. 申请；*vt*. 运用，应用

【搭配】apply for 申请；apply... to 将……应用于，涂，抹；apply oneself to (doing) sth. 致力于

【联想】application *n*. 申请；applicant *n*. 申请人

【例句】I want to apply for the job.

【译文】我想申请这项工作。

appoint [əˈpoint]　　　　　　*vt*. 任命，委派；约定

【搭配】appoint sb.（后面接名词）任命某人为……职

【联想】appoinment *n*. 任命，委派

【例题】To their surprise, she has been <u>nominated</u> as candidate for the Presidency.

　　　　A. recognized　　B. defined

　　　　C. appointed　　 D. promoted　　　C

【译文】出乎他们意料的是，她被提名为总统选举的候选人。

appreciate [əˈpriːʃieit]　　*vt*. 感激，感谢；评价；欣赏，赏识

【导学】后面接动名词，不接动词不定式，如：

appreciate（one's）doing。

【例句】 I appreciate President Castro's invitation for us to visit Cuba，and have been delighted with the hospitality we have received since arriving here.

【译文】 我感谢卡斯特罗主席邀请我们访问古巴。我们来到这里后受到了热情接待，使我一直沉浸在喜悦之中。

approach [ə'prəutʃ]　　　　*v.* 接近 *vt.* 处理；对待
　　　　　　　　　　　　　　 n. 靠近；方法；要求

【搭配】 approach to＝access to 接近

【例句】 They must change their institutional and legal approaches to water use.

【译文】 他们必须从制度和法规的方式上改变对水资源的使用。

appropriate [ə'prəupriət]　　　　*a.* 适当的，恰当的

【搭配】 be appropriate to 对……适合

【导学】 It's appropriate that... 从句中的谓语用原形或 should＋原形结构。

【例句】 It will be an indication that you are starting to get an appropriate amount of sleep at night.

【译文】 这将表明你正在进入夜间睡眠适量的时期。

approve [əˈpruːv]　　　　　　　*v.* 赞成，赞许，同意；
　　　　　　　　　　　　　　　　批准，审议，通过

【搭配】approve sth. 批准某事
　　　　approve of sth. 赞许、同意某事
　　　　approve of sb. doing sth. 同意某人做某事
【联想】approval *n.* 赞成，赞许
【例句】Mike Foster is trying to get Parliament to approve a new law.
【译文】迈克·福斯特正努力使国会通过一项新的法律。

Day 4

approximate [ə'prɒksimeit]　　　　　*a.* 大致的，近似的

archaeology [ˌɑːki'ɒlədʒi]　　　　　　　*n.* 考古学

architect ['ɑːkitekt]　　*n.* 建筑师；设计师；缔造者
【联想】architecture *n.* 建筑；建筑学

argument ['ɑːgjumənt]　　*n.* 争论，辩论；论点，依据
【联想】argue *vt. / vi.* 争论

arrange [ə'reindʒ]　　　*vt.* 整理，布置；安排，筹备
【搭配】arrange for sb. to do sth. 安排某人做某事
【联想】arrangement *n.* 安排

arrest [ə'rest]　　　　　　　　　*vt. /n.* 逮捕；扣留
【搭配】arrest sb. for 因……而逮捕某人
　　　　under arrest 被捕

arrogant ['ærəgənt]　　　　　　　*a.* 傲慢的，自大的
【联想】arrogancy *n.* 傲慢
【例句】Often these children realize that they know
　　　　more than their teachers, and their teachers

often feel that these children are arrogant, inattentive, or unmotivated.

【译文】 这些孩子常常觉得他们比老师知道的要多，老师们常常感到这些孩子自大、不用心或者缺乏学习动机。

artificial [ˌɑːtiˈfiʃəl]　　　　*a.* 人工的，人造的；人为的，做作的

【导学】 辨析 artificial, fake, false：artificial 指由人工制成的而非自然的；fake 指"伪造的，冒充的"；false 是指与真理或事实相反的，故意做假的。

【例句】 The colors in these artificial flowers are guaranteed not to come out.

【译文】 这些假花保证不会褪色。

aspect [ˈæspekt]　　　　　　*n.* 样子，面貌；方面

【联想】 respect *v.* 尊敬；inspect *v.* 视察；prospect *n.* 前景；expect *v.* 期望；perspective *n.* 洞察力

【例句】 Most national news has an important financial aspect to it.

【译文】 绝大多数的国内新闻都会涉及重要的金融信息。

assemble [əˈsembl]　　　　*vt.* 集合，集会；装配，组装
　　　　　　　　　　　　　　vi. 集会，聚集

【例题】 Everybody _____ in the hall where they

were welcomed by the Secretary.

A. assembled   B. accumulated

C. piled   D. joined

A

【译文】所有集聚在大厅的人都受到了部长的欢迎。

assembly [əˈsembli]   *n.* 集会，会议；装配，组装

【导学】辨析 assembly, conference, congress, convention，meeting：assembly 指"集会"；conference 指磋商或讨论的会议；congress 指代表大会，正式的代表举行会议讨论问题；convention 指某一团体或政党的正式会议；meeting 是常用词，表示"会议，大会"，也表示"会合，会面"。

aspire [əsˈpaiə]   *vi.* 追求，渴求，渴望（to, after）

【搭配】aspire to/after 渴望，向往

aspirin [ˈæspərin]   *n.* 阿司匹林

aspiration [ˌæspəˈreiʃən] *n.* 强烈的愿望，志向，抱负

【例句】But as useful as computers are，they are nowhere close to achieving anything remotely resembling these early aspirations for human-like behavior.

【译文】但是，尽管计算机非常有用，但它们离实现早期期望的类似人类行为的愿望还差之万里。

assassination [əˌsæsiˈneiʃən] 　　　　 *n.* 暗杀，刺杀

【联想】assassinate *vt.* 暗杀，行刺

【例句】Two members of a UN team investigating the February assassination of former Lebanese Prime Minister on Friday interviewed Lebanon's President.

【译文】周五，负责调查黎巴嫩前总理二月遭暗杀事件的两名联合国调查小组成员采访了黎巴嫩总统。

assert [əˈsəːt] *vt.* 宣称，断言；维护，坚持（权利等）

【例句】Why does the author assert that all things from American are fascinating to foreigners? Because they have gained much publicity through American media?

【译文】为什么作者断言美国所有的东西对国外人都有吸引力？因为它们通过美国的媒体已经获得了巨大的知名度吗？

assimilate [əˈsimileit] 　　　 *vt.* 吸收，消化；使同化
　　　　　　　　　　　　　　　　vi. 同化，融入

【例句】One of the reasons why children resemble their parents is that they assimilate the characteristics of their parents.

【译文】孩子长得像父母，其原因之一就是孩子吸取并同化了父母的各种特征。

assess [ə'ses]　*vt.* 估计，估算；评估，评价，评定

【联想】access *n.* 接近；excess *n.* 超额量；asset *n.* 资产

【导学】辨析 assess，estimate，evaluate：assess 指为征税估定（财产）的价值，确定或决定（某项付费，如税或罚款）的金额，评估某事物的价值、意义或程度；estimate 指估计，恰当地推测；evaluate 指确定……的数值或价值，对……评价，仔细地考察和判断。

asset ['æset]　*n.* 资产，财产；有用的资源，宝贵的人/物；优点，益处

【例题】He misled management by giving it the idea that the older and more experienced men were not an _____ but a liability.
A. assistance　　B. advantage
C. asset　　　　D. award　　　C

【译文】他认为年长者和有经验的人不是财产，而是累赘，这一观点误导了管理部门。

assign [ə'sain]　*vt.* 派给，分配；选定，指定（时间、地点等）

【联想】assignment *n.* （分派的）任务，（指定的）作业；分配，指派

【例题】In your first days at the school, you'll be

34

given a test to help the teachers to _____
you to a class at your level.

A. locate   B. assign
C. deliver   D. place   B

【译文】 在刚入学的几天里你会接受一项测试，以帮助老师为你选定一个适合你的水平的班级。

assist [əˈsist]   vi. 援助，帮助

【联想】 assistance n. 帮助，援助
【搭配】 assist in doing sth. 帮助做某事
assist sb. in doing sth. 帮助某人做某事
assist sb. to do sth. 帮助某人做某事
【例句】 The clerk assisted the judge by looking up related precedent.
【译文】 这位书记官协助那位法官查阅相关的判决先例。

associate [əˈsəuʃieit]   vt. 联系；联合 vi. 交往
n. 合作人，同事

【搭配】 associate...with 把……与……联系在一起
【联想】 association n. 协会，团体；交往；联合，合伙；
associate...with, link...to, relate...with/to,
combine/connect...with 把……与……联系在一起；have association with 与……交往
【例句】 What do you associate with such heavy snow?
【译文】 这样一场大雪，你有什么联想？

assume [əˈsjuːm]　　　　　　*vt.* 假定，设想；假装；承担

【联想】consume *v.* 消费；presume *v.* 推测；resume *v.* 重新开始；assumption *n.* 假定，设想；担任，承当；假装

【例句】Researchers conclude that any effect of money on happiness is smaller than most daydreamers assume.

【译文】研究者得出结论，金钱对幸福的影响程度要比大多数空想家假设的程度小。

assure [əˈʃuə]　　　　　　　*vt.* 使确信；向……保证

【导学】辨析 assure，ensure：两者皆意为"保证"，但用法有些区别，具体用法有 assure sb. that/assure sb. of；ensure that/ensure sb. against/from；assure/ensure sth.。

【联想】insure *v.* 保险，投保；assurance *n.* 保证

【例题】He was proud of being chosen to participate in the game and he _____ us that he would try as hard as possible.

　　A. assured　　　　B. insured

　　C. assumed　　　　D. guaranteed　　　　A

【译文】他为被选上参加比赛而感到骄傲，并且向我们保证他会尽其所能。

astonish [əs'tɒniʃ]　　　　　　　　*vt*. 使惊讶，使吃惊

【联想】astonishing *a*. 令人惊讶的
　　　　astonished *a*. 感到惊讶的
　　　　astonishment *n*. 惊讶

athlete ['æθli:t]　　　　　　　*n*. 运动员，运动选手

【联想】athletic *a*. 运动的，体育的，运动员的

atmosphere ['ætməsfiə]　　*n*. 空气；大气，大气层；
　　　　　　　　　　　　　　　气氛

ultimate ['ʌltimit] *a*. 最后的，最终的 *n*. 终极，顶点

【例句】The union leaders declared that the ultimate aim of their struggle was to increase pay and improve working conditions for the workers.

【译文】工会领导人宣称，他们斗争的最终目的是要增加工人工资和改善工人的工作条件。

undergo [ˌʌndə'gəu]　　　　　　*vt*. 经历，遭受

【搭配】undergo hardships/changes 经历苦难/变化

【导学】在英文中有许多以 under- 这个前缀开头的单词，多指"在……之下"。

【例句】Security programs should undergo actuarial review.

【译文】保障方案应经过精算评估。

undergraduate [ˌʌndəˈɡrædjuit]

n. 大学生，大学肄业生

【联想】undergraduate *n.* 本科生；postgraduate *n.* 研究生；Ph. student *n.* 博士生

understanding [ˌʌndəˈstændiŋ] *n.* 理解，理解力；谅解

a. 能体谅人的，宽容的

undertake [ˌʌndəˈteik] *vt.* 接收，承担；

约定，保证；着手，从事

【联想】undertaking *n.* 任务，项目；事业，企业；承诺，保证；殡仪业

【搭配】undertake to do/that 答应做

undertake an attack 发动进攻

undertake a great effort 做出巨大努力

uneasy [ʌnˈiːzi] *a.* 不安的，忧虑的

【联想】uneasiness *n.* 不安，焦虑

近义词为 nervous。

unfortunately [ʌnˈfɔːtʃənətli/ʌ] *ad.* 恐怕，不幸的是

union [ˈjuːnjən] *n.* 联合，结合，组合

协会，工会，联盟

unique [juːˈniːk]　　　　　　*a.* 唯一的，独一无二的

【搭配】be unique to... 对……来说是独一无二的

【例题】Speech is the _____ ability possessed only by human beings.

　　A. unique　　　　B. average

　　C. collective　　　D. single　　　　　　A

【译文】讲演是人类独有的能力。

universal [ˌjuːniˈvɜːsəl]　　　*a.* 宇宙的，全世界的；
　　　　　　　　　　　　　　　 普通的，一般的；通用的，万能的

【例句】Personal computers are of universal interest. Everyone is learning how to use them.

【译文】大家都对个人电脑感兴趣，每个人都在学习怎样使用它。

unlike [ˌʌnˈlaik]　　　　　　*a.* 不同的，不相似的
　　　　　　　　　　　　　　　 prep. 不像，和……不同

unusual [ʌnˈjuːʒuəl]　　　　*a.* 不平常的，稀有的；
　　　　　　　　　　　　　　　 例外的，独特的，与众不同的

upper [ˈʌpə]　　　　　　　　*a.* 上面的，上部的；较高的

【例句】A full moon was beginning to rise and peered redly through the upper edges of fog.

【译文】一轮满月开始升起，带着红色的光芒在雾气上沿朦胧出现。

upset [ʌp'set]　　　　*vt.* 弄翻，打翻；扰乱，打乱；使不安 *vi.* 颠覆

urban ['əːbən]　　　　*a.* 城市的，市内的

urge [əːdʒ] *v. /n.* 强烈希望，竭力主张；鼓励，促进

【搭配】urge sth. on 竭力推荐或力陈某事

【导学】在 urge that... 从句中，谓语动词用原形表示虚拟。

【例句】The urge to survive drove them on.

【译文】求生的欲望促使他们继续努力。

urgent ['əːdʒənt]　　　　*a.* 紧迫的；催促的

【例题】Since the matter was extremely _____, we dealt with it immediately.

A. tough　　　　B. tense

C. urgent　　　　D. instant　　　　C

【译文】既然事情比较紧急，我们马上处理吧。

usage ['juːzidʒ]　　　*n.* 用法，使用；惯用法，习语

utility ['juːtiliti]　　　*n.* 效用，实用；公用事业

【例句】The abstract shall state briefly the main

technical points of the invention or utility
model.

【译文】摘要应当简要说明发明或者实用新型的技术要点。

utilize [juːˈtilaiz]　　　　　　　*vt.* 利用，使用

utmost [ˈʌtməust]　　　　　　*a.* 最远的 *n.* 极限

utter [ˈʌtə]　　　　　　*a.* 完全的，彻底的，绝对的
　　　　　　　vt. 说，发出（声音）；说出，说明，表达

【搭配】utter one's thoughts/feelings 说出自己的想
法/感觉

【例句】What he is doing is utter stupidity!

【译文】他正在做的是完全愚蠢的事!

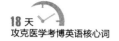
Day 5

atom ['ætəm]   *n.* 原子

【联想】 atomic *a*. 原子的，原子能的
     molecule *n*. 分子；particle *n*. 粒子
     electron *n*. 电子；nucleus *n*. 原子核

attack [ə'tæk] *n.* 袭击；攻击；抨击，非难；抑制；
发作，侵袭；（情感的）一阵突发；（病、虫
等的）损害 *v.* 袭击；攻击；（在战争等中使
用武器）进攻；抨击；非难；侵袭

【例句】 The school has come under attack for failing
     to encourage bright pupils.

【译文】 这所学校因未能鼓励聪明学生而受到非难。

attach [ə'tætʃ]   *vt.* 贴上，系上，附上；使依附

【搭配】 be attached to 喜爱，依恋，附属于
     attach importance to 重视……

【联想】 attachment *n*. 附件，依附

【例句】 I've attached my contact information in the
     recommendation letter.

【译文】 我在推荐信中附上了我的联系方式。

attain [ə'tein]   *vt.* 达到；取得

attendance [ə'tendəns]　　　　　n. 出席；出席的人数；
　　　　　　　　　　　　　　　　　　　伺候，照料

attendant [ə'tendənt]　n. 侍者，服务员；出席者；随从
　　　　　　　　　　　　　　　a. 出席的：随行的，伴随的

【导学】该词作为形容词不太被大家熟悉，但是形容
　　　　词的词意和用法也要掌握，如：attendant
　　　　problems 随之而来的问题。该词从动词
　　　　attend 派生出来，由于 attend 本身有多层意
　　　　思，所以要将该词与 attend 派生出来的其他
　　　　名词区分开来。

【例句】The Prime Minister was followed by five or
　　　　six attendants when he got off the plane.

【译文】首相从飞机上下来时有五六个随从跟着。

attitude ['ætitjuːd]　　　　　　　　n. 态度，看法

attraction [ə'trækʃən]　　　　　　n. 吸引；吸引力

【联想】attractive a. 有吸引力的；有魅力的，动人的

【例题】Niagara Falls is a great tourist _____,
　　　　drawing millions of visitors every year.

　　　　A. attention　　　B. attraction
　　　　C. appointment　　D. arrangement　　B

【译文】尼亚加拉大瀑布是一个著名的旅游景点，它每
　　　　年都会吸引数百万的游客。

attribute [ˈætribjuːt]   *n.* 属性，特征；

          [əˈtribjuːt]   *vt.* (to) 把……归因于

【搭配】attribute... to... 把……归因于……

【联想】contribute *v.* 贡献；distribute *v.* 分发

【例题】How large a proportion of the sales of stores in or near resort areas can be _____ to tourist spending?

     A. contributed   B. applied

     C. attributed   D. attached   C

【译文】在旅游点或者旅游点附近商店的销售中，有多大比例与旅游者的消费有关？

author [ˈɔːθə]   *n.* 作者

【导学】辨析 author，writer：author 指某作品的作者；writer 多指职业性作家。

authority [ɔːˈθeriti]   *n.* 权力，权威；权威人士；

                        (*pl.*) 当局

automatic [ɔːtəˈmætik]   *a.* 自动的

【例句】The factory is equipped with two fully automatic assembling lines, and the control room is at the center.

【译文】这座工厂配备两条全自动生产线，控制室就在正中央。

available [ə'veiləbl]　　　　　　*a.* 可利用的；可得到的

【导学】常做表语，做定语要放在所修饰词后面，如：These data are readily available. 这些资料很容易得到。

【例句】Humanity uses a little less than half the water available worldwide.

【译文】人类使用了全球可利用水资源的一小部分，不足一半。

average ['ævəridʒ]　　*a.* 平均的；典型的；正常的；普通的；平常的；一般的 *n.* 平均数；平均水平；一般水准 *v.* 平均为；计算出……的平均数

【例题】40 hours is a fairly average working week for most people.

【译文】对大多数人来说，每周工作 40 小时很正常。

avoid [ə'bvɔid]　　　　　　　　　　*vt.* 避免，逃避

【搭配】后面接动名词，avoid doing sth. 避免做某事。

【例题】They often try to avoid feeling unpleasant emotions, such as loneliness，worry，and grief.

【译文】他们经常尽量避免产生不愉快的情绪，例如孤独、担心和悲伤。

aware [ə'wɛə]　　　　　　　*a.* 知道的，意识到的

【搭配】be aware of 意识到

【例句】Coaches and parents should be aware, at all
times, that their feedback to youngsters can
greatly affect their children.

【译文】教练和父母要随时意识到他们的反应将会极大
地影响到他们的孩子。

awful ['ɔːful]   *a.* 糟糕的，极坏的，可怕的

【例句】She had put a good three miles between herself
and the awful hitchhiker.

【译文】她和那个吓人的旅行者之间保持了恰好三英里
的距离。

backlash ['bæklæʃ]   *n.* (对社会变动等的)
强烈抵制，集体反对

【例句】The government is facing an angry backlash
from voters over the new tax.

【译文】政府正面临选民对新税项的强烈反对。

bacteria [bæk'tiəriə]   *n.* (*pl.*) 细菌

【联想】bacterium *n.* 细菌（单数）

【例句】The bacteria which make the food go bad
prefer to live in the watery regions of the
mixture.

【译文】能使食物变坏的细菌更喜欢在有水的混合物区
域生存。

balance ['bæləns]　　　　　　　　　　*vt.* 使平衡
　　　　　　　　　n. 平衡；差额，结余；天平，秤

【搭配】off balance 不平衡

【例句】They throw out all ideas about a balanced diet for the grandkids.

【译文】他们将孙子、孙女的平衡饮食思想完全抛于脑后。

ban [bæn]　　　　　　　　　　*n. / vt.* 禁止，取缔

【例句】If the law is passed, wild animals like foxes will be protected under the ban in Britain.

【译文】如果这项法律通过了，像狐狸这样的野生动物在英国就将得到禁令的保护。

bare [beə]　*a.* 赤裸的，光秃的，空的；极少的，仅有的

【导学】辨析 bare，blank，empty，hollow，vacant：bare 表示赤裸的，没有通常或适当的覆盖物的；blank 指空白的，未填写的，没有字迹、图像或标记的；empty 指的是无人居住的，内无一物的，未载东西的，还指含义上空洞的；hollow 指中空的，凹的，挖空的；vacant 指空缺的，没有现任者或占有者的。

【例句】We'd better take the bare necessities.

【译文】我们最好只带极少的必需品。

barely ['beəli]　　　　　　　　　*ad.* 仅仅；几乎不能

【联想】seldom 几乎不；hardly 几乎不 rarely 几乎不

barrier ['bæriə]   *n.* 栅栏；障碍，屏障

【例句】Some people prefer the original English text whereas others feel a translation into their native language removes a barrier to understanding.

【译文】有人更喜欢英语原版，也有人觉得翻译成母语消除了理解上的障碍。

basically ['beisikəli]   *ad.* 基本地，根本地

basis ['beisis]   *n.* 基础，基底；基准；根据；主要成分（或要素）；（认识论中的）基本原则或原理

【搭配】on the basis of 根据，由于，以……为基础

【导学】该词复数形式为 bases

behave [bi'heiv]   *vi.* 举动，举止，表现

【联想】behaviour *n.* 行为，举止

【搭配】behave oneself 规规矩矩地

【例句】They still seemed to make people behave more honestly.

【译文】他们仍然好像能使人们举止坦诚。

benefit ['benifit]   *n.* 利益，恩惠
                    vt. 对（某人）有用，使受益 *vi.* 得益于

【联想】beneficial *a.* 有利的，有益的

【搭配】benefit from 受益于

bevarage [ˈbevərɪdʒ]   *n.* 酒水，饮料

biology [baiˈɔlədʒi]   *n.* 生物学

【例句】The girl shows a special interest in biology.

【译文】这个女孩对生物学表现出特殊的兴趣。

biomarker   *n.* 生物标志化合物

biomedical   *a.* 生物医疗的

bispectral   *a.* 双谱的

bound [baund]   *a.* 必定，约定；受约束；开往

【搭配】be/feel bound to do sth. 一定；必须；be bound for 准备起程开往……；在赴……途中

【例题】She seemed unwilling to acknowledge that this might not be wise and would be _____ to cause her husband concern.

　　A. obvious　　　B. indispensable

　　C. bound　　　D. doubtless   C

【译文】她看起来很不愿意承认这样是很不明智的，而且还会引起她丈夫的担心。

boundary [ˈbaundəri]   *n.* 界线，边界

breakthrough ['breikθru:]　　　*n*. 重大发现，"突破"

【导学】来自于词组 break through "突破"。常和 breakdown，outbreak 放在一起考辨析题。outbreak 意思是"（战争的）爆发，（疾病的）发作"。

【例句】While a full understanding of what causes the disease may be several years away, a breakthrough leading to a successful treatment could come much sooner.

【译文】尽管要完全理解这种疾病的病因还要好几年时间，但距离治疗方法的突破性进展已为时不远。

tackle ['tækl]　　　　　　　*vt*. 解决，处理

【例题】The local government leaders are making every effort to _____ the problem of poverty.

　　A. abolish　　　　B. tackle

　　C. remove　　　　D. encounter　　　B

【译文】当地政府领导正在努力解决贫困问题。

tactful ['tæktful]　　　*a*. 机智的；老练的，圆滑的

【例题】The doctor tried to find a <u>tactful</u> way of telling her the truth.

　　A. delicate　　　　B. communicative

　　C. skillful　　　　D. considerate　　　D

【译文】医生尽量用得体的方式告诉她真相。

talent ['tælənt] n. 天资；才能；人才

【搭配】have a talent for 对……有天赋
　　　　cultivate/develop one's talent 培养自己的才能

【例句】They also say that the need for talented, skilled Americans means we have to expand the pool of potential employees.

【译文】他们也指出对有才华的、技术熟练的美国人的需求，这意味着我们要挖掘员工的潜力。

target ['tɑːgit] n. 靶子，目标

【搭配】hit/miss the target 射中/未射中靶子

【例句】The Government has set the target for full implementation of whole-day primary schooling for 2007/2008.

【译文】政府已定下目标，将于2007～2008学年全面推行全日制小学。

tax [tæks] vt. 征税 n. 税款

【搭配】escape taxes 逃税；collect taxes 征税

【联想】tax-free a. 免税的 ad. 免税；taxpayer n. 纳税人

technician [tek'niʃ(ə)n] n. 技术员，技师，技工

technology [tek'nɔlədʒi]   *n.* 工业技术，应用科学

【联想】technological *a.* 技术的

teenager ['ti:nˌeidʒə]   *n.* (13～19岁的) 青少年

telehealth ['telihelθ]   *n.* 远程医疗

telescope ['teliskəup]   *n.* 望远镜

temper ['tempə]   *n.* 情绪，脾气

【搭配】be in a good/bad temper 心情好/不好；lose one's temper 发脾气，发怒

【例题】The violent _____ of his youth reappeared and was directed not only at the army，but at his wife as well.

A. impatience   B. character
C. temper   D. quality   C

【译文】他又犯了年轻时候的粗暴脾气，这次不仅针对的是部队，而且还有他的妻子。

temperament ['tempərəmənt]   *n.* 气质，性格

【例题】Whether a person likes a routine office job or not depends largely on temperament.

A. disposition   B. qualification
C. temptation   D. endorsement   A

【译文】一个人是否喜欢程式化的办公室工作很大程度上取决于性情。

temporary ['tempərəri]　　　　　*a.* 暂时的，临时的

【例句】 Their temporary mud huts with thatched roofs of wild grasses often only last six months.

【译文】 他们临时搭建的茅草屋顶的小泥屋通常只能维持6个月。

tempt [tempt]　　　　　*vt.* 引诱，勾引；吸引，引起……的兴趣

【导学】 近义词：lure，entice，fascinate，seduce，appeal to，induce，intrigue，incite，provoke，allure，charm，captivate，stimulate，move，motivate，rouse

【例句】 Your offer does not tempt me at all. Nothing can tempt me to leave my present position.

【译文】 你的建议一点也打动不了我的心，什么东西都不能诱使我离开现在的职位。

temptation [temp'teiʃən]　　　　　*n.* 引诱，诱惑；迷人之物，诱惑物

【例句】 It is not easy for us to resist temptation.

【译文】 对于我们来说，抵制诱惑是不太容易的。

terminate ['təːmineit]　　　　　*v.* 停止，(使) 终止

terminal ['təːminl]　　　　　*a.* 末端的，终点的；期末的；晚期的，致死的
　　　　　　　　　　　　　　　　n. 末端；总站；计算机终端

【搭配】terminal cancer 癌症晚期

terminal heart disease 心脏病晚期

【例句】His mom has a terminal illness.

【译文】他的母亲得了绝症。

therapy ['θerəpi]   *n.* 治疗，疗法

【联想】therapeutic *a.* 治疗的

threat [θret]   *n.* 威胁，危险现象

threaten ['θretn]   *vt.* 威胁，恐吓

【搭配】threaten sb. with/to do 用……威胁/威胁某
人要做

【联想】argue/persuade/talk sb. into doing sth. 说服某
人去做某事；cheat/trick sb. into doing sth. 哄
骗某人去做某事；force sb. into doing sth. 迫
使某人去做某事；frighten/scare/terrify sb.
into doing sth. 恐吓某人去做某事；reason sb.
into doing sth. 劝说某人去做某事

【例句】It will greatly threaten the security of this
country.

【译文】它将会极大地威胁这个国家的安全。

throat [θrəut]   *n.* 喉咙

【搭配】clear one's throat 清喉咙

have a bone in one's throat 难以启齿

tolerate [ˈtɔləreit]   *vt.* 忍受，容忍，容许

【联想】 tolerant *a.* 容忍的；tolerance *n.* 容忍

【例题】 Some old people don't like pop songs because
they can't _____ so much noise.
A. resist   B. sustain
C. tolerate   D. undergo   C

【译文】 一些老人不喜欢流行音乐，因为他们受不了那
么嘈杂的声音。

trace [treis]   *n.* 痕迹，踪迹 *vt.* 跟踪，查找

【搭配】 trace back to 追溯到

【例句】 Much of Chinese mythology is lost，and what
is not lost is scattered and difficult to trace.

【译文】 中国神话散佚很多，仅存的文献又很分散，难
以寻查。

tradition [trəˈdiʃən]   *n.* 传统，惯例

【联想】 traditional *a.* 传统的

tragedy [ˈtrædʒidi]   *n.* 悲剧；惨事，灾难

【联想】 tragic *a.* 悲剧的

trail [treil]   *n.* 痕迹，足迹 *vt.* 跟踪，追踪

Day 5

55

Day 6

calcium [ˈkælsiəm]   *n.* 钙

calculate [ˈkælkjuleit]   *vt.* 计算，推算；
估计，推测；计划，打算

【联想】calculation *n.* 计算；calculator *n.* 计算器

【例句】The tuition is too high to be calculated.

【译文】学费太高，无法计算了。

calorie [ˈkæləri]   *n.* 卡（热量单位）

【例句】I would like to have a cup of black coffee. I am counting my calories at the moment.

【译文】我想要一杯不加糖和奶的咖啡（黑咖啡）。我目前正在控制所摄取的热量。

cancel [ˈkænsəl]   *vt.* 取消，撤销；删去

【联想】cancellation *n.* 取消，删除

【例句】All flights having been canceled because of the snowstorm, they decided to take the train.

【译文】因为暴风雪，所有的航班都取消了，他们决定坐火车。

cancer [ˈkænsə]   *n.* 癌

【联想】 cancerous a. 癌症的

candidate [ˈkændidit]　　n. 候选人；报考者；求职者

【例句】 A second language isn't generally required to get a job in business, but having language skills gives a candidate the edge when other qualifications appear to be equal.

【译文】 掌握第二门语言通常不是在贸易方面找到一份工作的条件，但是有语言方面的技能则能使候选人在其他条件同等的情况下比其他人具有更大的优势。

capability [ˌkeipəˈbiliti] n. 能力，才能；性能，容量

【联想】 capable a. 能干的，有能力的，有才能的

【搭配】 have the capability of 有……的才能
beyond/above one's capability 超过某人的能力范围

【联想】 have the ability to do, have the capacity for doing/to do 有能力做

capacity [kəˈpæsiti]　　　　n. 容量，容积；能力；能量；接受力

【例句】 The memory capacity of bees means they can distinguish among more than 50 different smells to find the one they want.

【译文】 蜜蜂的记忆力意味着它们能在50多种不同的味

Day 6

道中找到它们想要的那种。

capture [ˈkæptʃə]   *vt.* 捕获，捉拿；夺得，攻占

【例句】The decline in moral standards—which has long concerned social analysts—has at last captured the attention of average Americans.

【译文】被社会学家一直关注的道德滑坡问题，最终引起了美国大众的关注。

carbon [ˈkɑːbən]   *n.* 碳

carbonhydrate [ˌkɑːbəuˈhaidreit]   *n.* 碳水化合物

cardiac [ˈkɑːdiæk]   *a.* 心脏的；心脏病的
                          n. 心脏病患者；强心剂；健胃剂

【联想】cardiologist *n.* 心血管医生

cardivascular [ˌkɑːdiəuˈvæskjələ(r)]   *a.* 心血管的

career [kəˈriə]   *n.* 生涯，经历；专业，职业

【例句】A lateral move that hurt my feelings and blocked my professional progress, promoted me to abandon my relatively high profile career.

【译文】一次侧面的打击伤害了我的感情，阻碍了我事业的发展，使我放弃了我那份引人注目的工作。

carefree ['kɛəfriː] *a.* 快乐的，无忧无虑的

caring ['kɛəriŋ] *a.* 关心人的，人道的，有同情心的

carrier ['kæriə] *n.* 搬运人；携带者；运载工具

casual ['kæʒuəl] *a.* 随便的；偶然的；临时的

【例句】 Friendships among Americans tend to be casual.

【译文】 美国人之间的友谊往往是比较随意的。

catastrophe [kə'tæstrəfi] *n.* 大灾难，大祸

【例题】 Losing his job was a financial <u>catastrophe</u> for his family.

　　A. calamity　　　B. accident

　　C. frustration　　D. depression　　　A

【译文】 整个家庭因为他的失业而陷入了财政危机。

【导学】 近义词：disaster, calamity, mishap, mischance, misadventure, failure, fiasco, misery, accident, trouble, casualty, misfortune, infliction, affliction, contretemps, stroke, havoc, ravage, wreck, fatality, grief, crash, devastation, desolation, avalanche, hardship, blow, visitation, ruin, reverse, emergency, scourge, cataclysm, convulsion, debacle, tragedy, adversity，bad luck，upheaval

catalog ['kætəlɒg]　　　　*n.* 目录 *vt.* 将……编入目录

category ['kætigəri]　　*n.* 种类，类别；(逻) 范畴

caution ['kɔːʃən]　　　　　　*n.* 谨慎，小心；警告

【联想】 cautious *a.* 谨慎的，小心的
【搭配】 do sth. with caution 谨慎小心地做
　　　　caution sb. against/about sth. 警告某人某事
【例句】 Others viewed the findings with caution，
　　　　noting that a cause-and-effect relationship
　　　　between passive smoking and cancer remains
　　　　to be shown.
【译文】 其他人谨慎地看待这些发现，因为他们注意到在
　　　　被动吸烟和癌症之间的因果关系仍然有待观察。

cervical ['sɜːvɪkl]　　　　　　　*a.* 子宫颈

challenge ['tʃælindʒ]　　　　　　*n.* 挑战，挑战书；
　　　　艰巨任务，难题 *vt.* 向……挑战

【搭配】 challenge sb. to do sth. 向某人挑战做某事
　　　　challenge sb. to sth. 向某人挑战某事

change [tʃeindʒ] *vt.* 改变，变更，变革；交换，更
　　　　迭，替换；把……变成……(into) *n.* 改变，
　　　　变化；找回的零钱；调换 (口味)；换衣服

【联想】changeable *a.* 可交换的

character [ˈkærɪktə]　*n.* 性格，品质；特性，特征；
人物，角色；（书写或印刷）符号，（汉）字

【导学】辨析 character, nature, personality：
character 指性格、品性、人格，尤指是非
观念、品德等；nature 指性格、天性、气
质等的总称，与生俱来的，也指事物的性
质或人类的通性；personality 指个性、个
人魅力，强调感情因素。

characteristic [ˌkærɪktəˈrɪstɪk]　*a.* 特有的，独特的
n. 特征，特性

【导学】辨析 characteristic, feature, property,
quality：characteristic 指人、物或抽象的特
点或特征，是识别他人或他物的明显标志；
feature 指显著的非常突出的特点，具有足
以引人注目的部分或细节，常用于生理、自
然条件、物品等；property 性质、特征，通
常指事物的基本特征；quality 指个人的品
行、品质。

characterize [ˈkærɪktəraiz]　*vt.* 描绘……的特性，
刻画……的性格

【例句】Our society is characterized with the "knowledge

economy".

【译文】我们的社会以"知识经济"为特征。

cheat [tʃiːt]　　　　　*vt.* 哄骗，骗取 *vi.* 作弊，欺诈
　　　　　　　　　　　　　　n. 欺骗，骗子

【搭配】cheat sb. (out) of sth. 骗取某人的某物
　　　　cheat sb. into the belief that 哄骗某人相信

【导学】辨析 cheat, deceive：cheat 指用诡计欺骗，骗取；deceive 表示误导，使……相信不真实的情况，做出错误的判断。

【例题】When I caught him _____, I stopped buying things there and started dealing with another shop.

　　A. cheating　　　　B. cheat
　　C. to cheat　　　　D. to be cheating　　A

【译文】我抓住他在欺骗后，我停止在那里买东西而开始在另一家商店购物。

chemical [ˈkemikəl]　　　　　　　　*a.* 化学的
　　　　　　　　　n. 化学制品/产品/物质/成分

【例句】The carbon dioxide would then be extracted and subjected to chemical reactions.

【译文】二氧化碳然后被提取出来，并将其进行化学反应。

chemist [ˈkemist]　　　　　　*n.* 化学家，药剂师

chemotherapy [ˌkiːmə(u)'θerəpi]   *n.* 化疗

cigar [si'gɑː]   *n.* 雪茄烟

circular ['səːkjulə]   *a.* 圆形的；循环的

circulate ['səːkjuleit]   *v.* （使）循环，（使）流通

【例题】This local evening paper has a _____ of twenty-five thousand.

    A. number   B. contribution

    C. circulation   D. celebration   C

【译文】当地晚报的发行量为 25 000 份。

circumstance ['səːkəmstəns]

                n. (*pl.*) 情形，环境；条件

【搭配】under the circumstances 在这种情况下，情况既然如此；under/in no circumstances 在任何情况下都不（放在句首要倒装）

【导学】辨析 circumstances, environment, setting, surroundings：circumstances 指某事或某动作发生时的情况，形势；environment 指周围的状况或条件，可以是自然环境，也可以是社会环境，可以是物质上的，也可以是精神上的；setting 指某一情形的背景或环境；surroundings 指围绕物，周围的事物。

【例题】We have been told that under no circumstances _____ the telephone in the office
for personal affairs.

    A. may we use   B. we may use

    C. we could use   D. did we use   A

【译文】我们被告知，在任何情况下，我们都不允许为
了私人的事情而使用办公室的电话。

transaction [trænˈzækʃən] *n.* 交易，事务，处理事务

【搭配】conduct transaction 进行交易

【例句】As they bought and sold assets, they had
trouble remembering that each transaction
could impact their monthly cash flow.

【译文】当他们买卖资产时，总是难以记住每笔交易都
会对他们的每月现金流量产生影响。

transcend [trænˈsend]   *vt.* 超出，超越
                   （经验、理性、信念等的）范围

【导学】近义词：exceed, overreach, overrun, over-
step, surpass, excess

transfer [trænsˈfəː] *vt.* 迁移，调动；换车；转让，过户
        [ˈtrænsfə(r)] *n.* 迁移，调动；换车；转让，过户

【搭配】transfer sth. from... to 转移，调任，换乘

【例句】Transfer research results into commodities

according to market rules.

【译文】将研究成果按市场规律转换成商品。

transform [træns'fɔːm] *vt.* 转换，变形；变化，变压

【联想】change... into，turn... into 由……变成

【例题】The twentieth century has witnessed an enormous worldwide political, economic and cultural _____.

A. tradition   B. transportation

C. transmission   D. transformation   D

【译文】20世纪见证了世界范围内的政治、经济和文化各方面的巨大转变。

transistor [træn'zistə]   *n.* 晶体管（收音机）

transit ['trænsit]   *n.* 通行，运输

【例句】We observed the transit of Venus across the sun last night.

【译文】我们昨晚观测到金星凌日。

transition [træn'ziʃən] *n.* 转变，变迁，过渡（时期）

【导学】近义词：shift，passage，flux，passing，development，transformation，turn

【例句】The transition from childhood to adulthood is always a critical time for everybody.

【译文】从童年到成年的过渡对每个人来说都是一个关

键的时期。

transplant [træns'plɑːnt]　*vt.* 移栽，移种（植物等）；
移植（器官）；使迁移，使移居
['trænsplɑːnt]　　　　　　　*n.*（器官的）移植

【导学】注意该词的名词形式同样也可以做定语。

【例句】When any non-human organ is transplanted into a person, the body immediately recognizes it as foreign.

【译文】当任何非人类的器官移植到人体内，身体很快便能识别出它是异物。

translation [træns'leiʃən]　　　　　　　*n.* 翻译

transmit [trænz'mit]　　　　*vt.* 传送，传输，传达，
传导，发射 *vi.* 发射信号，发报

【联想】transmission *n.* 传输，传达

【搭配】transmit a match live 实况转播比赛

【例题】Some diseases are _____ by certain water animals.

　　　　A. transplanted　　B. transformed
　　　　C. transported　　D. transmitted　　D

【译文】一些疾病是通过某种水栖动物传播的。

transparent [træns'pɛərənt]　　　　　　*a.* 透明的

【联想】transparency *n.* 透明度

transport [træns'pɔːt]　　　　　　*vt.* 运输，运送

　　　　　　['trænspɔːt]　　　　　　　*n.* 运输，运送

【联想】 transportation *n.* 运输，运输系统

【例句】 Additional social stresses may also occur because of the population explosion or problems arising from mass migration movements—themselves made relatively easy nowadays by modern means of transport.

【译文】 由于人口猛增或大量人口流变动（现在交通运输工具使大量人口流动变得相对容易）所引起的各种社会问题也会对社会造成新的压力。

treatment ['triːtmənt]　　　*n.* 待遇，对待；治疗，疗法

trial ['traiəl]　　　　　　　　　*n.* 试验；审判

【搭配】 be on trial 实验性地；在受审

typical ['tipikəl]　　　　　　　*a.* 典型的，有代表性的；独有的，独特的

【搭配】 be typical of 代表性的，典型的

Day 7

cite [sait]   *vt.* 举（例），引证，引用

civil ['sivl]   *a.* 市民的，公民的，国民的；民间的；
                                民事的，根据民法的；文职的

【例句】He left the army and resumed civil life.

【译文】他离开了军队，恢复了平民生活。

civilian [si'viljən]   *a.* 平民的，民用的，民众的

civilization [ˌsivilai'zeiʃən]   *n.* 文明，文化

【联想】civilize *vt.* 使开化，使文明，教化

【例句】Both civilization and culture are fairly mod-
          ern words, having come into use during the
          19th century by anthropologists.

【译文】文明和文化都是相当时髦的词汇，是人类学家
          在 19 世纪开始使用的词汇。

claim [kleim] *n.*（根据权利提出）要求，要求权，主
          张，要求而得到的东西 *vt.*（根据权利）要求，
                                认领，声称，主张，需要

【导学】辨析 claim, proclaim：claim 一般指声称对某

物的拥有权；proclaim 常为官方正式宣布。

clarify ['klærifai]　　　　　　　*vi.* 澄清，阐明 *vt.* 使明晰

【导学】辨析 clarify，clear，clean：clarify 指使清晰
或易懂，详细阐明，澄清混乱或疑惑；clear
指去除物体或障碍，使明确，使明朗，去除
困惑、疑问或模棱两可，也指天空变晴；
clean 指扣除，清除，去除垃圾或杂质。

classic ['klæsik]　　　　　　　*n.* 杰作，名著 *a.* 第一流的

classical ['klæsikəl]　　　　　　　　　*a.* 经典的，古典的

classify ['klæsifai]　　　　　　　　　　*vt.* 分类，分级

【联想】classification *n.* 分类，分级

【例句】Stereotypes seem unavoidable, given the way
the human mind seeks to categorize and
classify information.

【译文】鉴于人类大脑进行信息的归类和分类的方法，
刻板印象似乎是不可避免的。

climate ['klaimit]　　　　　　　　*n.* 气候；风气，思潮

【联想】climatic *a.* 气候的，与气候有关的

clinic ['klɪnɪk]　　　　　　　*n.* 诊所；（医院的）门诊部；
　　　　　　　　　　　　　　门诊时间；会诊时间；私人诊所
　　　　　　　　　　　　　　专科医院；门诊治疗部；临床实习

collaborate [kə'læbəreit]　　　　　　*v.* 合作，协作

【联想】collaboration *n.* 合作，协作

colleague ['kɔli:g]　　　　　　　　*n.* 同事，同僚

【导学】辨析 colleague，partner：colleague 指同事、
　　　　同行、职员或学院教工的同僚之一；partner
　　　　指伙伴，同伙，或在一项活动或一个涉及共
　　　　同利益的领域内与另一人或其他人联合或有
　　　　联系的人，尤指企业合作人、配偶、舞伴、
　　　　搭档等。

combine [kəm'bain]　　　　　　*v.* 结合，联合，化合

【搭配】combine with 与……联合（化合、结合）
【联想】combination *n.* 结合，联合

comment ['kɔment]　　　　　　*n. /v.* 解说，评论

【搭配】comment on/upon 评论，谈论，对……提意见
【例句】The range of news is from local crime to
　　　　international politics, from sport to business
　　　　to fashion to science, and the range of
　　　　comment and special features as well, from
　　　　editorial page to feature articles and
　　　　interviews to criticism of books, art, theatre
　　　　and music.
【译文】新闻的范围从当地的犯罪到国际政治，从体育

到商业，到时尚，到科学。评论和特写的范围
也是从社论到专栏文章，以及对书籍、艺术、
戏剧和音乐的评论。

commerce [ˈkɒmə(ː)s] *n.* 商业，贸易

【联想】commercial *a.* 商业的，商务的 *n.* 商业广告

communicate [kəˈmjuːnikeit] *vt.* 传达；交流；通信
  vi. 传达，传播

【搭配】communicate with 和……联系，和……通信
  communicate sth. to sb. 把……传达给某人

【联想】communication *n.* 通讯；通信；交际，交流；传达，传送

community [kəˈmjuːniti] *n.* 社区

【例句】A hero has a story of adventure to tell and community will listen to.

【译文】英雄总有冒险的故事可讲，而公众又愿意去听。

comparable [ˈkɒmpərəbl] *a.* 可比较的，比得上的

【搭配】be comparable with 可与……相比的，与……类似的；be comparable to 可与……比拟的，与……匹敌的

【例句】Nevertheless, children in both double-income and "male breadwinner" households spent comparable amount of time interacting with their parents.

【译文】然而，在双收入家庭和父亲为收入来源的家庭中，孩子和父母互动的时间相当。

comparative [kəm'pærətiv]　　　*a*. 比较的，相当的

comparison [kəm'pærisn]　　　　*n*. 比较；对比

【搭配】in comparison with 与……比较
　　　　by comparison 比较起来

compassionate [kəm'pæʃənit]　　*a*. 有同情心的，
　　　　　　　　　　　　　　　　　　深表同情的

【联想】comgpassion *n*. 同情

【例题】I have never seen a more caring, _____ group of people in my life.
　　　　A. emotional　　　B. impersonal
　　　　C. compulsory　　D. compassionate　　D

【译文】在我一生中还从没见过比这群人更体贴更富有同情心的。

compensate ['kɔmpənseit]　　　　*vt*. 补偿，偿还，
　　　　　　　　　　　　　　酬报（for）；给……付工钱；赔偿

【搭配】compensate sb. for 因……而赔偿某人
　　　　compensate for 弥补

【联想】compensatory *a*. 补偿性的，弥补性的

【例句】To compensate for his unpleasant experiences

he drank a little more than how much was good for him.

【译文】为了借酒消愁，他喝得有点过了头。

compensation [ˌkɔmpen'seiʃən]　　　*n.* 补偿，赔偿

【导学】该词属于常考词汇，经常出现在阅读和词汇部分。

【例句】The insurance company paid him $10,000 in compensation after his accident.

【译文】事故之后，保险公司支付给他一万美元作为赔偿。

complain [kəm'plein]　　　*vi.* 抱怨，诉苦，申诉

【搭配】complain to sb. of/about sth. 向某人抱怨某事
complain of doing sth. 抱怨做某事

【联想】complaint *n.* 抱怨，怨言；控告

【导学】complain 后面只接 that 从句做宾语，不直接跟 sb. 或 sth. 做宾语。

complement ['kɔmplimənt]　　　*n.* 补足；余数；补语

【联想】complementary *a.* 补足的，补充的

【例句】Movie directors use music to complement the action on the screen.

【译文】电影导演运用音乐与屏幕上的情节相配合。

complicated ['kɔmplikeitid]　　*a.* 错综复杂的，难懂的

【联想】complicate *vt.* 使复杂化，使混乱，使难懂

【例句】This is too complicated a matter to settle all by myself.

【译文】这事太复杂，我一人难以对付。

complication [ˌkɔmpli'keiʃ(ə)n]   *n.* 错杂；
新增的困难，新出现的问题；并发症

【例题】His broken arm healed well, but he died of pneumonia which followed as a _____.

　　A. complement   B. compliment

　　C. complexion   D. complication   D

【译文】他的断臂愈合得很好，但最终死于肺炎这一并发症。

conceal [kən'si:l]   *vt.* 隐瞒，隐藏，隐蔽

【搭配】conceal sth. from sb. 对某人隐瞒某事物

【例句】John's mindless exterior concealed a warm and kindhearted nature.

【译文】约翰漫不经心的外表掩盖了他热情、善良的本性。

concentrate ['kɔnsentreit]   *vt.* 集中；聚集；浓缩
vi. 集中，专心

【搭配】concentrate on/upon 集中在，专心于

【联想】concentration *n.* 专注，专心；集中，浓度

【例题】Rejecting the urging of his physician father to study medicine，Hawking chose to _____ on math and theoretical physics.

A. impose B. center

C. overwork D. concentrate   D

【译文】霍金拒绝了做内科医生的父亲让他学习医药的要求，选择了专攻数学和理论物理。

safeguard ['seifgɑːd]　　　　v. 保护，保障，捍卫
　　　　　　　　　　　　　　n. 安全设施，保护措施

sake [seik]　　　　　　　　n. 缘故，理由

【搭配】for the sake of 为了

【例句】We should continue to integrate theory with practice，study for the sake of application，and acquire a better understanding of the theory of Marxism.

【译文】我们要继续理论联系实际，学以致用，提高马克思主义的理论水平。

sanction ['sæŋkʃən]　　　　n. 认可，许可，批准；
　　　　　　　　　　　　　　支持，赞成；制裁，处罚

satellite ['sætəlait]　　　　n. 卫星，人造卫星

【搭配】launch a satellite 发射卫星

【例句】We receive television pictures by satellite.

【译文】我们通过人造卫星接收电视图像。

satisfactory [ˌsætis'fæktəri]　　　　　*a.* 令人满意的

【例句】The plan is almost satisfactory in every way.

【译文】这个计划几近完美。

saving ['seiviŋ]　　　*n.* 储蓄；(*pl.*) 储蓄金，存款

【搭配】deposit one's savings 存款

scaffold ['skæfəuld]　　　　　　　　　　*n.* 断头台

scale [skeil]　　　　　*n.* 标度，刻度 (*pl.*) 天平，
　　　　　　　　　　　　天平盘；标尺，比例尺；音阶

【搭配】on a large scale 大规模地

【例句】It may be possible for large-scale change to occur
without leaders with magnetic personalities, but
the pace of change would be slow.

【译文】缺乏独特个人魅力的领导者也有可能推动大规
模的变革，但变化的进度可能会慢一些。

scan [skæn]　　　　　　　　　*n. / v.* 浏览；扫描

【例句】He scanned *Time* magazine while waiting at
the doctor's office.

【译文】在医生的诊所候诊时，他翻阅了《时代》周刊。

scarcely ['skɛəsli]   *ad.* 几乎不；勉强

【搭配】scarcely... when 一……就

【联想】scarece *a.* 稀少的，罕见的

scare [skɛə]   *vt.* 惊吓，使恐惧 *vi.* 惊慌，惊恐

scatter ['skætə]   *vi.* 撒，驱散，散开；
                                        散布，散播 *vt.* 分散，消散

【导学】辨析 scatter, disperse, spread：scatter 指由
       于外力使人或物杂乱地向不同的方向散开或
       散播；disperse 指有目的地、安全地解散或
       彻底散开，范围较前者广；spread 指在表层
       分散，也可指疾病、谣言的传播。

【例句】I hate to scold，but you mustn't scatter your
       things all over the place.

【译文】我不想训斥你，但你不该总把东西到处乱丢。

scenario [sə'nɑːriəu]   *n.* 脚本；方案；设想；预测；
                                    （电影或戏剧的）剧情梗概

【例句】Let me suggest a possible scenario.

【译文】我来设想一种可能出现的情况。

scratch [skrætʃ]   *v.* 搔，抓，扒；勾销，删除
                                    n. 搔，抓，抓痕

【搭配】scratch a living 勉强维持生活

【例句】 The scratch on your hand will soon be well.

【译文】 你手上的划伤不久就会好。

scream [skri:m]   *vi*. 尖叫

secondary ['sekəndəri]   *a*. 第二的，中级的；
                                            次要的，次等的

sedantary ['sedntri]   *a*. 久坐不动的，静止的

segregate ['segrigeit]   *v*. 隔离并区别对待
（不同种族、宗教或性别的人）；（使）隔离

【联想】 segragation *n*. 种族隔离；隔离

shallow ['ʃæləu]   *a*. 浅的；浅薄的，肤浅的
                                            n. (*pl.*) 浅滩，浅处

shortcoming ['ʃɔːtkʌmiŋ]   *n*. 短处，缺点

shortly ['ʃɔːtli]   *ad*. 立刻，马上

shrink [ʃriŋk]   *vi*. 起皱，收缩；退缩，畏缩

【例句】 Shrinking landfill space, and rising costs for
burying and burning rubbish are forcing local
governments to look more closely at recycling.

【译文】 掩埋式垃圾处理场可占用的空间逐渐缩小，同
时，掩埋和燃烧垃圾的成本却在增长，这迫使

当地政府更加重视回收利用。

signal ['signl]　　*n.* 信号，暗号 *v.* 发信号，打暗号

【联想】signature *n.* 签字，签名

significant [sig'nifikənt]　　　　*a.* 重大的；重要的；
意味深长的

【联想】significance *n.* 意义，含义；重要性

simulate ['simjuleit]　　*vt.* 模仿，模拟；假装，冒充

【例句】We used to use this trick in the army to simulate illness.

【译文】我们在军队服役时常用这一伎俩装病。

situated ['sitjueitid]　　　　　　*a.* 位于，坐落于

【搭配】be situated at/in/on 位于

【例句】The housing development must be situated near public transportation.

【译文】住房开发必须位于靠近公共交通的地方。

skeptical ['skeptikəl]　　　　　　*a.* 表示怀疑的

【导学】和它的近义词一起记忆：doubtable，suspicious。

【例句】Ignorant people were skeptical of Columbus' theory that the earth is round.

【译文】那时，无知的人对于哥伦布的地球是圆形的理

论表示怀疑。

slaughter ['slɔːtə]　　　　　*n.* 屠杀，杀戮；屠宰

【导学】表示杀的词还有：butcher 屠宰，屠杀；massacre 残杀，集体屠杀；carnage（尤指在战场上的）残杀，大屠杀，流血；assassinate 暗杀，行刺。

【例句】I could not stand to watch them slaughter the cattle.

【译文】看到他们在屠杀那群牛，我受不了。

soak [səuk]　　　　　　　*v.* 浸湿，浸透

soar [sɔː, sɔə]　　　*vi.* 高飞，翱翔；高涨，猛增

social ['səuʃəl]　　　*a.* 社会的；社交的，交际的

【例句】Social studies is the study of how man lives in societies.

【译文】社科课程是研究人们怎样在社会中生活的学科。

solar ['səulə]　　　　　　*a.* 太阳的，日光的

【搭配】solar system 太阳系

sophisticated [sə'fistikeitid]　　*a.* 先进的，复杂的；精密的；老于世故的

【例句】The British in particular are becoming more

sophisticated and creative.

【译文】特别是英国人变得更加成熟和有创造力。

specialist ['speʃəlist]　　　　　　　　　　*n.* 专家

【搭配】a specialist in/on 在……方面的专家

specialize ['speʃəlaiz]　　　　　*vi.* 专攻，专门研究

【搭配】specialize in 专攻

specially ['speʃəli]　　*ad.* 特别地，特地；格外地

species ['spi:ʃi:z]　　　　　*n.* (物) 种，种类

specific [spi'sifik]　　　　　　　*n.* 特效药，细节
　　　　　　　　　　a. 详细而精确的，明确的；特殊的，
　　　　　　　　　　特效的；(生物) 种的

【联想】specifically *ad.* 特定地，明确地

specify ['spesifai]　　　　　　*vt.* 指定，详细说明

specimen ['spesimn]　　　　　　*n.* 样本，标本

【搭配】collect specimens 采集标本

Day 8

confidence [ˈkɔnfidəns]　　　 n. 信任，信心；秘密

【搭配】in confidence 秘密地；with confidence 充满
自信地；have confidence in 对……有信心

confident [ˈkɔnfidənt]　　　 a. 确信的，有自信的

【搭配】be/feel confident in/of 确信某事

【联想】be/feel certain of, be/feel sure of, be convinced
of, have confidence in 确信某事

【例句】He is confident that scientists can block transmission of malaria to humans.

【译文】他确信科学家能够阻止疟疾向人类的传播。

confidential [ˌkɔnfiˈdenʃəl]　　　 a. 秘密的，机密的；
表示信任（或亲密）的

confirmation [ˌkɔnfəˈmeiʃən]　　　 n. 确定，确立，
证实；确认，批准

【联想】confirm vt. 证实，进一步确定，确认；批准

【例题】Wainwright found confirmation that Morrell
gave Hitler antibiotics as a precaution in a
recent translation of Morrell's own diary.

[2010]

【译文】 温顿特最近在翻译莫雷尔的私人日记时确认，莫雷尔给希特勒注射了抗生素预防针。

confront [kən'frʌnt]   *vt.* 使面对，使遭遇

【联想】 confrontation *n.* 面对；对峙（抗）；对质

【例题】 *China Daily* never loses sight of the fact that each day all of us _____ a tough, challenging world.

A. encounter   B. acquaint

C. preside   D. confront   D

【译文】 《中国日报》从未忘记这样一个事实，即我们所有人每天都面临着一个艰难而又有挑战性的世界。

conserve [kən'sɜ:v]   *vt.* 保存，保护；节约，节省

【导学】 conserve, protect, reserve, preserve：conserve 指保护从而使其不受损失或伤害，也指节约，谨慎或节省地使用，避免浪费；protect 指保护使免于受到损坏、攻击、偷盗或伤害；reserve 指收藏保留，如用于将来使用或某个特殊的目的，也指"预订，预约"；preserve 意为"保存，保持，收藏"，指保护某物不受破坏，使之完好无损。

【例句】 If no one owns the resource concerned, no one has an interest in conserving it or

Day 8

fostering it: fish is the best example of this.

【译文】 如果相关的资源没有主人，就不会有人有兴趣去保存或培养它：鱼就是这方面的最好例证。

considerable [kən'sidərəbl]　　　*a.* 相当的；可观的

【例题】 The visit of Lian Zhan to the mainland received _____ attention at this time.
A. significant　　B. considerable
C. enormous　　D. numerous　　　　　B

【译文】 连战此次访问大陆引起了相当大的关注。

considerate [kən'sidərit]　　　*a.* 考虑周到，体谅的，体贴的

【例题】 It is _____ of you to turn down the radio while your sister is still ill in bed.
A. considerable　　B. considerate
C. concerned　　D. careful　　　　　B

【译文】 你妹妹生病卧床的时候你能把收音机的音量调小，真是考虑周到。

consideration [kən,sidə'reiʃən]　　*n.* 考虑；要考虑的事；体贴，关心

【搭配】 take... into consideration 顾及……，考虑到……

【例题】 Although architecture has artistic qualities, it

must also satisfy a number of important practical _____ .

A. obligations B. regulations
C. observations D. considerations D

【译文】虽然建筑具有艺术特质，但是它也要满足一些重要的实际需求。

considering [kən'sidəriŋ] *prep*. 就……而论，照……说来；鉴于

consolidate [kən'sɔlideit] *v*. 加固，巩固

【导学】该词属于常考词汇，尤其出现在词汇部分。考生要注意常用的相关同义词：solidify（使……凝固，使……团结，巩固），strengthen（加强，巩固），unify（使联合，统一）。

【例句】Consolidate and develop socialist relations characterized by equality, unity and mutual assistance among all ethnic groups for common prosperity and progress.

【译文】巩固和发展平等、团结、互助的社会主义民族关系，实现各民族共同繁荣和进步。

constant ['kɔnstənt] *a*. 不断的，持续的；始终如一的；坚定的，忠实的；恒定的，经常的

【导学】辨析 constant, continual, continuous：constant

表示连续发生的，在性质、价值或范围上持久不变的，始终如一的；continual 表示有规律地或经常地发生，强调中间有间断的连续；continuous 表示不间断的连续。

【例句】 The newly-designed machine can help the room maintain a constant and steady temperature.

【译文】 这种新设计的机器能够帮助房间保持一个稳定不变的温度。

consult [kənˈsʌlt]　　　　*vt*. 请教，咨询；查阅；就诊
　　　　　　　　　　　　vi. 商量；会诊

【搭配】 consult... about... 向······讨教某事；consult with... about... 跟某人商量某事

【导学】 辨析 consult，consult with：consult 指"向······请教或咨询"，或指"参考，查阅"；consult with 指"磋商，交换意见"。

consultant [kənˈsʌltənt]　　　　　　　　　*n*. 顾问

【导学】 辨析 consultant，guide：consultant 指提供专家意见或专业意见的人；guide 指在方法或道路上引导或指导另一人的人，或在行为等方面堪称他人楷模的人。

【例题】 I think we need to see all investment _____ before we make an expensive mistake.

　　　A. guides　　　　　　B. entrepreneurs

C. consultants   D. assessors

【译文】 我认为我们必须拜访所有的投资顾问以免犯下代价昂贵的错误。

contact [ˈkɒntækt]　　　　　*n. /vt.* 接触，联系，交往

【联想】 container *n.* 容器，集装箱

【搭配】 be in (out of) contact with 与……有（失去）联系

【联想】 keep in touch with sb. 与某人保持联系

contaminate [kənˈtæmineit]　　　　　*vt.* 弄脏，污染

【例句】 Now a paper in *Science* argues that organic chemicals in the rock come mostly from contamination on earth rather than bacteria on Mars.

【译文】 最近《科学》上的一篇文章宣称：岩石中的有机化学物质主要来自地球本身的污染，而并非来自火星上的细菌。

contract [ˈkɒntrækt]　　　　　*n.* 契约，合同，包工
　　　　　[kənˈtrækt]　　　　　*v.* 收缩；感染；订约

【搭配】 enter into/make a contract (with sb.) (for sth.) （与某人）（为某事）订立和约；sign a contract 签订合同；contract with 与……订合同

contrast [ˈkɒntræst]　　　　　　　*v. /n.* 对比，对照

【搭配】in contrast with/to 和……形成对比（对照）

contrast A with B 把 A 与 B 对照

【例题】Preliminary estimation puts the figure at around $110 billion, _____ the $160 billion the president is struggling to get through the Congress.

A. in proportion to　B. in rely to

C. in relation to　　D. in contrast to　　D

【译文】预先估算的款项在 1100 亿美元左右，而总统正尽力通过议会获得 1600 亿。

controversial [ˌkɒntrəˈvɜːʃəl]　　*a.* 争论的；引起争论的；被议论的；可疑的

【例题】The idea of correcting defective genes is not particularly <u>controversial</u> in the scientific community.

A. inevitable　　　B. applicable

C. disputable　　　D. incredible　　C

【译文】在科学界，对于矫正缺陷基因的想法并没有什么争议。

convention [kənˈvenʃən]　　　　*n.* 习俗，惯例；大会，会议；公约

【联想】conventional *a.* 普通的，常见的；习惯的，

常规的

【搭配】break established conventions 打破成规；sign a convention of peace with a neighbouring country 与邻国签订一项和平协定

【例题】The North American states agreed to sign the <u>agreement</u> of economical and military union in Ottawa.

A. convention   B. conviction

C. contradiction   D. confrontation   A

【译文】北美各国同意在渥太华签署经济军事联盟协议。

cooperate [kəu'ɔpəreit]   *vi.* 合作，协作，相配合

【搭配】cooperate with sb. in doing sth. 与某人合作做某事

【例句】The British cooperated with the French in building the new craft.

【译文】英、法两国合作制造这种新式飞船。

coordinate [kəu'ɔːdinit]   *v.* (使) 协调，调整；(使) 互相配合

【搭配】coordinate with each other 互相配合

corporate ['kɔːpərit]   *a.* 公司的；法人组织的；社会团体的；共同的；自治的

【联想】corporation *n.* 公司，团体

countdown ['kauntdaun]   *n.* 倒数计秒

counter ['kauntə]   *n.* 计算器，计数器，计算者；
柜台；筹码 *ad. / a.* 相反地（的）

counterpart ['kauntəpɑːt]   *n.* 对等的人；副本

【导学】该词属于常考词汇，主要出现在词汇选择和阅读部分。其中 counter 原指"柜台"，可想象成顾客和服务生面对面的场景，转义为"相对的"。

【例句】Your right hand is the counterpart of your left hand.

【译文】你的右手是你左手的相对物。

crash [kræʃ]   *v. / n.* 摔坏，坠毁

【导学】辨析 crash, crush, smash: crash 指"坠毁"，碰撞中造成的突然损毁; crush 指"压碎"，把（石头或矿石等）挤压、捣碎或碾成小碎块或粉末; smash 指"打碎"，或突然地、大声地、猛力地把某种东西毁成碎片。

【例题】After our computer network _____ for the third time that day, we all went home.

A. crashed   B. collided

C. smashed   D. fell

【译文】那天在我们的电脑网络系统第三次崩溃之后，

我们都回家了。

create [kri'eit] *vt*. 创造，创作；产生；制造，建立

【联想】creative *a*. 有创造力的，创造性的

credential [krə'denʃl]   *n*. 资质
                                   vt. 提供证明书（或证件）

crime [kraim]   *n*. 罪，罪行，犯罪

【联想】criminal *a*. 犯罪的，刑事的 *n*. 罪犯，刑事犯

criterion [krai'tiəriən]   *n*. 标准，准则

【导学】该词经常用于指代各类赛事的评分标准，常见的近义词：rule（准则），standard（标准），regulation（规则）等。

【例句】The most important criterion for assessment in this contest is originality of design.

【译文】这次比赛最重要的评判标准就是设计的原创性。

critic ['kritik]   *n*. 批评家，评论家

critical ['kritikəl]   *a*. 批评的，批判的；危急的，紧要的

【搭配】be critical of 挑剔，不满

【例句】We are at a critical point in our nation's

history.

【译文】我们现在正处于我们国家历史中的一个关键时刻。

criticize [ˈkritisaiz]　　　　　　　　*vt.* 批评，评论

【联想】criticism *n.* 批评，评论

crucial [ˈkruːʃiəl, ˈkruːʃəl]　　　　*a.* 关键的，决定性的

cultivate [ˈkʌltiveit]　　　　*vt.* 耕作，栽培，养殖；
　　　　　　　　　　　　　　　　培养，陶冶，发展

【例句】They have enough money and leisure time to cultivate an interest in the arts.

【译文】他们有足够的金钱和空闲时间来培养艺术方面的兴趣。

culture [ˈkʌltʃə]　　　　　　　　*n.* 文化，文明；教养

spectacular [spekˈtækjulə]　　　　　　*a.* 壮观的

speculate [ˈspekjuleit]　　　　*vi.* 思索，推测；投机

【搭配】speculate about/on/over 推测；speculate in 投机

【例句】We are living in the here and can only speculate about the hereafter.

【译文】我们生活在现在，只能预测未来。

spiritual ['spiritjuəl]   *a.* 精神（上）的，心灵的

spokesman ['spəuksmən]   *n.* 发言人

stable ['steibl]   *a.* 安定的，稳定的

【联想】stabilize *vt.* 使稳定，使稳固

【例句】People guess that the price of oil should remain stable for the rest of the year.

【译文】人们估计在今年剩下的日子里油价会保持稳定。

standpoint ['stændpoint]   *n.* 立场，观点

【搭配】maintain/alter one's standpoint 坚持/改变立场

starve [stɑːv]   *vt.* 使饿死 *vi.* 饿得要死

【搭配】starve for 渴望，急需

statement ['steitmənt]   *n.* 陈述，声明

【搭配】confirm a statement 证实某一说法

statistic [stə'tistik]   *n.* 统计数值

status ['steitəs]   *n.* 地位，身份；情形，状况

【例题】China believes that nuclear-weapon states should respect the status of nuclear-weapon-free zones and assume corresponding obligations.

【译文】中国认为，核武器国家应尊重无核武器区的地

位并承担相应的义务。

steady ['stedi]　　　　*a*. 稳定，不变；稳固，平稳；坚定，扎实 *v*. (使) 稳定

stimulate ['stimjuleit]　　　　*vt*. 刺激，激励，使兴奋

【搭配】stimulate sb. into/to sth. 鼓励某人做

【例题】An important property of a scientific theory is its ability to _____ further research and further thinking about a particular topic.
A. stimulate　　　　B. renovate
C. arouse　　　　　D. advocate　　　A

【译文】科学理论最重要的特性在于它能够推进某个特定主题的进一步研究和思考。

stimulus ['stimjuləs]　　　　*n*. 刺激物

【导学】stimulus 后通常与介词 to 搭配。

【例句】During the first two months of a baby's life, the stimulus that produces a smile is a pair of eyes.

【译文】婴儿出生的头两个月，刺激他微笑的是别人的眼睛。

strategy ['strætidʒi]　　　　*n*. 战略；策略

【搭配】adopt/apply/pursue a strategy 采取策略

【例句】Meanwhile，we will also carry out the open strategy of Going Global and encourage qualified companies with competence to make overseas investment.

【译文】 同时，我们还要实施"走出去"开放战略，鼓励有条件有实力的企业到境外投资办厂。

substance ['sʌbstəns]　　　　　*n*. 物质；实质，本质；要旨，大意

【搭配】 in substance 大体上是，从本质上说
【例句】 Water consists of various chemical substance.
【译文】 水由各种不同的化学物质构成。

subtract [səb'trækt]　　　　　*vt*. 减，减去

【例句】 He could add and subtract, but hadn't learned to divide.
【译文】 他会做加减法，但还没有学会除法。

suicide ['sjuisaid]　　　　　*n*. 自杀

【搭配】 commit suicide 自杀

superficial [sju:pə'fiʃəl] *a*. 表面的；肤浅的，浅薄的

surgery ['sə:dʒəri]　　　　　*n*. 外科，外科手术

【联想】 surgical *a*. 外科（医术）的；外科用的，外科手术的

surveillance [sə:'veiləns] *n*. 监控；（对犯罪嫌疑人或可能发生犯罪的地方的）监视

Day 8

sustain [səs'tein]　　　　*vt.* 支撑，撑住；经受，忍耐

【联想】sustainable *a.* 可以忍受的，足可支撑的，养得起的

sympathetic [ˌsimpə'θetik]　　　*a.* 同情的，共鸣的

【搭配】be sympathetic to... 对……表示同情

【联想】sympathize *vt.* 同情，怜悯，共鸣
sympathy *n.* 同情，同情心；赞同，同感
sympathize with sb., show sympathy towards sb., feel/express sympathy for/with sb., have sympathy for sb. 同情

symptom ['simptəm]　　　　*n.* 症状，征候

【搭配】have/show the symptoms of a cold 有感冒的症状

synthetic [sin'θetik]　　*a.* 合成的，人工的；综合的
n. 人工制品（尤指化学合成物）

【例句】The store now offers 531 varieties of synthetic fabrics, all Chinese-made.

【译文】这个店现在出售 531 种合成纤维，全部都是中国生产的。

systematic(al) [ˌsisti'mætik]　　　*a.* 系统的；
有计划的，有步骤的；有秩序的，有规则的

Day *9*

dairy ['dεəri]　　　　　　　*n.* 牛奶场；乳品店；乳制品

【联想】milk *n.* 牛奶；cream *n.* 奶油；cheese *n.* 乳
　　　酪；powdered milk *n.* 奶粉；butter *n.* 黄油

dash [dæʃ]　　　　　　*vt.* 猛掷，猛撞 *vi.* 猛冲
　　　　　　　　　　　　n. 猛冲，短跑，破折号

【例句】The boat was dashed against the rocks.

【译文】那船猛地撞到礁石上。

data ['deitə]　　　　　*n.* (datum 的复数) 资料，材料

【导学】做主语时，谓语可以是单数，也可以是复数。

【例句】There are more than 2.5 million workers who
　　　need help, according to Labour Department
　　　data.

【译文】根据劳动部的数据，有 250 多万名工人需要
　　　帮助。

database ['deitəbeis]　　　　　　　　　　*n.* 数据库

【导学】该词在历年考题中均出现在阅读部分。需要
　　　注意的是，data 来源于 datum，表达复数概
　　　念。

【例句】This information is combined with a map database.

【译文】这一信息同地图数据库有效地结合在一起。

deadline ['dedlain]　　　*n*. 最后期限，截止交稿日期

deadly ['dedli]　　　*a*. 致命的，致死的；极有害的

【导学】辨析 deadly, fatal, mortal：deadly 意为"可能致死的"（likely to cause or able to produce death），表示能够或可能引起死亡，但不一定有导致死的结果；fatal 意为"导致死亡的"（causing or resulting in death），多指已经或将导致死亡，强调死亡是不可避免的；mortal 意为"死亡的"，指未能永存。

【例句】It was the worst tragedy in maritime history, six times more deadly than the Titanic.

【译文】这是航海史上一次空前的灾难，所造成的损失是泰坦尼克号的六倍之多。

debate [di'beit]　　　*vt*. 争论，辩论

【例句】We debated the advantages and disadvantages of filming famous works.

【译文】关于把名著拍成电影的优点和缺点，我们进行了辩论。

Debilitate [di'biliteit]　　*vt*. 衰弱；（使身心）衰竭；虚弱；削弱（国家、机构）的力量

decade ['dekeid]   *n.* 十年

【例句】 For the past decade or so, practical courses, such as computer and business, have gained tremendous development on collage campuses.

【译文】 过去十年来，实用性课程，诸如计算机和商业课程已在大学校园中得到极大的发展。

decay [di'kei]   *n.* 衰退，腐烂 *v.* 衰退，腐烂

【例句】 Dr. Li of the U. S. Department of Agriculture, has found that oranges can be prevented from decaying by the use of certain chemicals containing sulfur compounds.

【译文】 美国农业部的李博士发现，使用某种含硫的化合物能防止橘子腐烂。

declaration [ˌdeklə'reiʃən] *n.* 宣布，宣告；声明；申报

decrease [di:'kri:s]   *v. / n.* 减少，减小

dedicate ['dedikeit]   *vt.* 奉献

【例句】 I want to see all of us dedicate ourselves to the principles for which we fought.

【译文】 我希望看到所有的人献身于我们为之奋斗的原则中去。

degeneracy [di'dʒenərəsi]   *n.* 堕落，退化，退步

degrade [di'greid]　　　　*v.* 分解，降级，使受屈辱

deliberate [di'libəreit]　　*a.* 故意的；深思熟虑的

　　　　　　　　　　　　　　　v. 仔细考虑

【例句】Sometimes the messages are conveyed through deliberate, conscious gestures.

【译文】有时，信息是通过故意的、下意识的手势表达的。

delicate ['delikit]　　　*a.* 纤弱的，娇嫩的，易碎的；优美的，精美的，精致的；微妙的，棘手的；灵敏的，精密的

【例句】Delicate plants must be protected from cold wind and frost.

【译文】娇弱的植物必须妥善保护，以避免风霜的侵袭。

democracy [di'mɔkrəsi]　　*n.* 民主，民主制；民主国家

【联想】democratice *a.* 民主的，有民主精神（作风）的

demonstrate ['demənstreit]　　*vt.* 表明；论证；演示

　　　　　　　　　　　　　　　　　　vi. 示威

【搭配】demonstrate against 示威反对

【例句】History has demonstrated that countries with different social systems can join hands in meeting the common challenges.

【译文】历史表明，不同社会体制的国家能够联手迎接共同的挑战。

depress [di'pres]   *vt*. 压抑；降低

【例题】 When business is _____, there is usually an obvious increase in unemployment.

A. degraded   B. depressed

C. reduced   D. lessened   B

【译文】当经济下滑，失业率就会有明显的上升。

depressant [di'presnt]   *n*. 抑制剂

a. 有镇静作用的；使消沉的

depression [di'preʃən] *n*. 不景气，萧条；沮丧，消沉

【例题】 Many people lost their jobs during the business _____.

A. despair   B. decrease

C. desperation   D. depression   D

【译文】经济不景气时，许多人都失去了工作。

deprive [di'praiv]   *vt*. 剥夺，夺去，使丧失

【搭配】 be deprived of 被剥夺

【例句】 And it made him determined to do something for convicts and slaves and for all who were oppressed and deprived of their liberty.

【译文】这促使他下定决心去为了罪犯和奴隶，为了所

有受压迫、被剥夺了自由的人们做点儿力所能
及的事。

desperate ['despərit]   *a.* 绝望的，危急的；
不顾一切的，铤而走险的

【例句】 Thousands of Mexicans arrive each day in this
city, desperate for economic opportunities.

【译文】 每天都有成千上万的墨西哥人到达这个城市，
渴望获得发财的机会。

destination [ˌdesti'neiʃən]   *n.* 目的地，终点；
目的，目标

detail ['diːteil, di'teil]   *n. / vt.* 细节；说情
枝节，琐事；详述，详谈

【搭配】 in detail 详细地
【联想】 detailed *a.* 详细的

deteriorate [di'tiəriəreit]   *v.* 恶化，变坏，蜕变

【例句】 Some scientists are dubious of the claim that
organisms deteriorate with age as an inevitable outcome of living.

【译文】 有机组织随着年龄的增长而退化是不可避免
的自然生理现象，对这一论断有科学家持怀
疑态度。

deterioration [di₋tiəriəˈreiʃən]   *n.* 变坏，退化；堕落

【联想】 deteriorate *vi.* 恶化，变坏

【例题】 The recent <u>deterioration</u> in the economy is of great concern to the government.

    A. depression   B. deficiency

    C. degeneration   D. deformity   C

【译文】 近期的经济恶化成了政府的关注点。

detrimental [₋detriˈmentl]   *a.* 有害的，不利的

【例题】 The chemical was found to be <u>detrimental</u> to human health.

    A. toxic   B. immune

    C. sensitive   D. allergic   A

【译文】 这种化学品被发现对人类健康有害。

devastate [ˈdevəsteit]   *v.* 使荒芜，破坏；压倒

【例题】 It will be a <u>devastating</u> blow for the patient, if the clinic closes.

    A. permanent   B. desperate

    C. destructive   D. sudden   C

【译文】 如果关闭门诊，对病人将是毁灭性的打击。

【导学】 近义词：ravage, desolate, waste; overwhelm, confound, crush

diabetes [₋daiəˈbiːtiːz]   *n.* 糖尿病

diagnose [ˈdaiəgnəuz]　　　　　　*v.* 诊断；判断

【例句】One of my neighbors caught a bad cold and went to his doctor, who diagnosed his cold as SARS.

【译文】我的一个邻居感冒得很厉害，去看病时被医生诊断为非典型性肺炎。

diagnosis [ˌdaiəgˈnəusis]　　　　*n.* 诊断；调查分析

【导学】diagnosis 复数形式为 diagnoses。

diarrhea [ˌdaiəˈriːə]　　　　　　　*n.* 腹泻

racial [ˈreiʃəl]　　　　　　　　*a.* 人种的，种族的

【例句】There is no racial discrimination to be felt in this city.

【译文】在这个城市里感觉不到种族歧视。

racism [ˈreisizəm]　　*n.* 种族主义；种族歧视（意识）

radiate [ˈreidieit]　　　　　*v.* （使）闪光，发光
　　　　　　　　　　　　　　　（使）辐射；（使）显出，流露

【例句】In the darkness, his eyes seemed to radiate some inner strength.

【译文】黑暗中，他的双眼似乎流露出某种内在的力量。

radical ['rædikəl]　　　　　　*a.* 基本的，重要的；
　　　　　　　　　　　　　　　　　激进的，极端的

radiologist [ˌreidi'ɔlədʒist]　　*n.* 放射科医生；
　　　　　　　　　　　　　　　　　X 光科的医生

rampant ['ræmpənt]　　*a.* 泛滥的；猖獗的；疯长的
【例句】Unemployment is now rampant in most of
　　　　Europe.
【译文】在欧洲的大部分地区，失业问题难以控制。

random ['rændəm]　　　　*a.* 随机的；任意的，随便的
　　　　　　　　　　　　　　n. 偶然的（或随便的）行动（或过程）
【搭配】at random 随便的，任意的
【例句】When a psychologist does a general experi-
　　　　ment about the human mind，he selects peo-
　　　　ple at random and asks them questions.
【译文】当心理学家做关于人类心理的普遍实验时，他
　　　　通常会随机选择人来问一些问题。

range [reindʒ]　　　　　　*n.* 范围，距离，领域；
　　　　　　　　　　　　　　　排列，连续，（山）脉
【搭配】range from... to... 从……到……不等
【例句】Your Bluetooth Wireless Headset can commu-
　　　　nicate with other Bluetooth devices within a

range of approximately 10 meters (33 feet).

【译文】 你的无线蓝牙耳机可在约 10 米（33 英尺）范围内与其他蓝牙设备进行通讯。

rank [ræŋk]　　　　　　*n.* 排，行列；等级，地位
　　　　　　　　　　　　　vt. 评价，分等，归类

【例题】 New York _____ second in the product of apples, producing 85,000,000 pounds this year.

　　　A. ranked　　　　B. occupied

　　　C. arranged　　　D. classified　　　A

【译文】 纽约今年的苹果产量排名第 2 位，总产量达到 8 500 万磅。

rare [reə]　　　　　　　*a.* 稀有的，难得的，珍奇的；
　　　　　　　　　　　　　　　　　稀薄的，稀疏的

【导学】 辨析 rare, scarce：rare 指罕见的、稀奇的物品；scarce 指寻常物的短缺。

【例句】 It is a rare treasure of historical records.

【译文】 这是史上罕见的史料珍品。

rarely [ˈreəli]　　　　　*ad.* 稀少，很少，难得

【例题】 San Francisco is usually cool in the summer, but Los Angeles _____.

　　　A. is rarely　　　　B. is scarcely

C. hardly is   D. rarely is   D

【译文】 在夏天，旧金山通常很凉爽，但是在洛杉矶就极少这样了。

rash [ræʃ]   *a.* 轻率的，鲁莽的

【例句】 I'm not very happy about our rash decision.

【译文】 我不很赞成我们的草率决定。

rate [reit]   *n.* 速率，比率；等级；价格，费用
                             vt. 评级，评价

【搭配】 at any rate 无论如何，至少

【导学】 辨析 rate，ratio：rate 意为"速率，速度"，一般用词，既可指速度又可指比率，如 survival rate（成活率）；ratio 意为"比率，比例"，指两个同类数互相比较，其中一个数是另一个数的几倍或几分之几，如 4：3。

【例题】 Recycling waste slows down the rate _____ which we use up the Earth's finite resources.
A. in   B. of
C. with   D. at   D

【译文】 废物再利用减缓了我们消耗地球有限资源的速度。

ratio ['reiʃiəu]   *n.* 比率，比

rational ['ræʃənl]   *a.* 理性的，合理的

【例句】Respecting persons, therefore, means to respect them as rational creatures.

【译文】因此，尊重他人也就是尊重他们为理性人。

raw [rɔ:]　　　　　　　*a.* 生的，未煮熟的；未加工过的

react [ri'ækt]　　　　　　*vi.* 反应，起作用

【搭配】react to 对……做出反应

reaction [ri(:)'ækʃən]　　　*n.* 反应；反作用（力）

【搭配】reaction to 对……的反应

【例题】It was difficult to guess what her _____ to the news would be.

　　　A. reaction　　　　B. impression

　　　C. comment　　　　D. opinion　　　A

【译文】很难猜测她对这个新闻的反应。

readily ['redili]　　　　　*ad.* 容易地，乐意地

realistic [riə'listik]　　　*a.* 现实的，现实主义的；逼真的

reality [ri(:)'æliti]　　　　*n.* 现实，实际；真实

【搭配】in reality 实际上，事实上

realm [relm]　　　　*n.* 王国，国度；领域，范围

reap [ri:p]　　　　　　*v.* 收割，收获

【例句】 Anyone clever enough to modify this information for his own purposes can reap substantial rewards.

【译文】 任何一个足够聪明的人出于个人目的修改这项资料，就能从中获取丰厚的酬劳。

rear [riə]　　　　*n.* 后部，尾部 *a.* 后方的，背后的
　　　　　　　　　　　　　　　　　vt. 饲养；抚养

【搭配】 at the rear of 在······的后部

reasonable ['riːznəbl]　*a.* 合理的，讲理的；公道的

【例句】 This statement is a reasonable conclusion looking at world politics and economics.

【译文】 看看世界的政治与经济就可以说这是个合理的断言。

recall [ri'kɔːl]　　　　*vt.* 回想；叫回；收回

【例题】 I remember seeing him years ago, but I cannot _____ where it was.

　　A. remind　　　　B. recognize
　　C. recall　　　　 D. memorize　　　C

【译文】 我记得几年前看到过他，但是具体的位置我已经记不清了。

reciprocal [ri'siprəkəl]　　　*a.* 相互的，互惠的

【例题】 The two countries will assign counter-drug

officials to their respective embassies on a
_____ basis.

A. fundamental   B. similar

C. reciprocal   D. reasonable   C

【译文】这两个国家将在互惠的基础上，互派缉毒官员
到各自的大使馆。

recreation [rekri'eiʃ(ə)n]   *n.* 娱乐，消遣

region ['ri:dʒən]   *n.* 地区，区域；范围

【联想】regional *a.* 区域的

【例句】The bacteria which make the food go bad
prefer to live in the watery regions of the
mixture.

【译文】能使食物变坏的细菌更喜欢在混合物的含水区
域生存。

Day *10*

diet [ˈdaiət]   *n.* 饮食，食物

【联想】dietary *a.* 饮食的

【搭配】be/go on a diet 节食

disabled [disˈeib(ə)ld]   *a.* 残疾的，残废的

disadvantage [ˈdisədˈvɑːntidʒ]
                          n. 不利，不利条件；缺点，劣势

disappointed [ˌdisəˈpɔintid]   *a.* 失望的

disaster [diˈzɑːstə]   *n.* 灾害，灾难，灾祸

discard [disˈkɑːd]   *vt.* 丢弃，舍弃，抛弃

discharge [disˈtʃɑːdʒ]   *v. / n.* 卸（货），解除，
                          排出；释放，允许离开；放电

discriminate [disˈkrimineit]   *vt.* (between) 区分，
                          辨别；(against) 歧视

【导学】搭配介词：from "将……同……区分开
来"，between "区分，辨别"，against "歧

111

视，排斥"。

【例句】However, paradoxically, just recently a group of black parents filed a lawsuit in California claiming that the state's ban on IQ testing discriminates against their children by denying them the opportunity to take the test.

【译文】然而荒谬的是，就在最近，加州的一群黑人家长一纸诉讼，状告地方所颁布的智商测试禁令歧视黑人小孩，剥夺了孩子们参加考试的机会。

disseminate [di'semineit]　　　　*vt.* 散布，传播

disgrace [dis'greis]　　　　*n.* 耻辱，丢脸的人（或事）
　　　　　　　　　　　　　　　　　v. 玷污

dismay [dis'mei]　　　　*n.* 失望，气馁，惊愕
　　　　　　　　　　　　　　vt. 使失望，使惊愕

【例句】I was dismayed at Professor Smith's comment on my paper.

【译文】听到史密斯教授对我的论文的评价，我感到沮丧。

dismiss [dis'mis]　　　　*vt.* 不再考虑；免职，解雇，开除；解散

【例题】The company was losing money, so they had to <u>lay off</u> some of its employees for three months.

A. owe   B. dismiss

C. recruit   D. summon

【译文】公司正在亏损，因此他们不得不让部分员工停工3个月。

dispatch/despatch [dis'pætʃ]   *v.* 分派特定任务

n. 派遣

displace [dis'pleis]   *vt.* 取代，替代；

迫使……离开家园，使离开原位

【例句】Television has displaced motion picture as America's most popular form of entertainment.

【译文】电视取代了电影的地位，成了美国最为普遍的娱乐方式。

distract [dis'trækt]   *vt.* 使……分心，使分散注意力

【例句】Although we tried to concentrate on the lecture, we were distracted by the noise from the next room.

【译文】尽管我们试图将注意力集中在讲座上，但隔壁房间传来的噪声还是让我们分了神。

disturb [dis'tə:b]   *vt.* 扰乱，妨碍；打扰，使不安

【例句】Please don't disturb me while I'm working.

【译文】请不要在我工作时打扰我。

disturbance [dis'təːbəns]　　　 *n.* 动乱；骚扰，干扰；（身心）失调

【例句】This disturbance would have occurred sooner or later.

【译文】这场风波迟早要来。

domain [də'mein]　　 *n.* （活动、思想等）领域，范围；领地，势力范围

【例句】If you do not confirm this Internet domain change with your ISP, you will not be able to send or receive E-mail.

【译文】如果不与ISP确认该Internet域的更改，你将无法收发电子邮件。

dominate ['dæmineit]　　　　 *vt.* 支配，统治，控制；高出于，居高临下 *vi.* 居支配地位，处于最重要的地位

【联想】domination *a.* 支配的，统治的，居高临下的；显性的

【例题】For the past two years, Audi cars have _____ Germany's Touring Car Championship.

　　　A. dominated　　　B. conquered

　　　C. determined　　　D. contested

【译文】 在过去的两年里，奥迪汽车一直是德国房车锦标军赛的冠军。

donate [dəu'neit]　　　　　　　*v*. 捐赠，馈赠

【例句】 President donated thousands of books to the local library and visited the local schools with his wife.

【译文】 总统向当地的图书馆捐赠了几千本图书，并和夫人一起参观了当地的几所学校。

dramatic [drə'mætik]　　　　*a*. 戏剧的，戏剧性的；引人注目的 *n*. (*pl*.) 戏剧，戏曲

drawback ['drɔːbæk]　　*n*. 困难，缺点，不足之处

【例题】 Is it true that is the major <u>drawback</u> of the new medical plan?

　　A. defect　　　　　B. assistance
　　C. culprit　　　　　D. triumph　　　A

【译文】 那真的是新医疗计划的主要缺点吗？

duplicate ['djuːplikeit]　　　　　　　*vt*. 复制
　　　　　　['duːplikət]　　　　　*n*. 复制品，副本

【例句】 The problem, the scientists say, is that AI has been trying to separate the highest, most abstract levels of thought, like language and mathematics, and to duplicate them with logical，step-by-step programs.

【译文】科学家们认为，问题在于 AI 一直试图将最高级、最抽象的思维层次分离开来，如语言和数学思维，并利用逻辑程序逐步将这些思维复制。

durable ['djuərəbl]   *a*. 耐久的

【例句】They are often more comfortable and more durable than civilian clothes.

【译文】它们常常比平时穿的衣服更舒适耐用。

duration [djuə'reiʃən]   *n*. 持续，持续时间

eczema ['eksimə]   *n*. 湿疹

economical [ˌiːkə'nɔmikəl]   *a*. 节俭的，节省的，
                                       经济的

【导学】辨析 economic, economical：economic 表示经济的或与之有关的，经济学的或与之有关的；economical 表示节俭的，不浪费或不挥霍的，节约的，通过高效率的运作和削减不必要的性能来节省费用的。

economy [i(ː)'kɔnəmi]   *n*. 经济，经济制度；
                                       节约，节省

educate ['edju(ː)keit]   *vt*. 教育，培养，训练

【例句】An educator must first educate himself.

【译文】教育者必须自己先受教育。

effective [i'fektiv]　　　　　*a.* 有效的，生效的

【导学】辨析 effective，efficient，valid：effective 表示有效的，具有预期或先见效果的，既强调产生满意的效果，又注重不浪费时间、精力等因素，因此往往带有"有效率的"意味；efficient 意为"有能力的；高效率的"；valid 表示（法律上）有效的，正当的，或在一段时间、某种情况下有效的。

【例句】A proven method for effective textbook reading is the SQ3R method.

【译文】经过证明的一种有效的阅读课本的方法是 SQ3R 方法。

elaborate [i'læbərət]　　　　　*a.* 精细的，详尽的
　　　　　　[i'læbəreit]　　　　　*v.* 详细描述

【例句】They had created elaborate computer programs to run the system.

【译文】他们创造了非常精细的计算机程序来运行这个系统。

elastic [i'læstik]　　　　　*n.* 橡皮圈，松紧带
　　　　　　　　　　　　　　　a. 有弹性的，弹力的；灵活的，可伸缩的

【例句】Our plans are still very elastic.

【译文】我们的计划仍然是有弹性的。

elevate ['eliveit] *vt.* 提升……的职位，提高，改善；
使情绪高昂，使兴高采烈；举起，使上升

【导学】近义词：hoist, heave, tilt, levitate, raise；
advance, upgrade, further, promote

【例句】Second, will male-dominated companies elevate women to higher-paid jobs as they elevate men?

【译文】其二，男性一统天下的公司会像他们提拔男性一样提拔女性到高薪岗位吗？

eliminate [i'limineit] *vt.* 消灭，除去，排出

【例句】She has been eliminated from the swimming race because she did not win any of the practice races.

【译文】她已被取消了参加游泳比赛的资格，因为她在训练中没有得到名次。

embrace [im'breis] *vt.* 抱，拥抱；包括，包含；
包围，环绕

emigrate ['emigreit] *vi.* 移居外国，移民

emit [i'mit] *vt.* 发出，发射；散发（光、热、气味等）

emotion [i'məuʃən]   *n.* 情感，情绪

【导学】 emotion，feeling，passion：emotion 一般指比较强烈、深刻且能感动人的感情或情绪，多含精神上的反应，如爱、惧、哀、乐等；feeling 泛指人体的一切感觉、情绪和心情；passion 意为"激情"，指往往由于正确的判断受其影响而表现出强烈的或激烈的情绪，有时不能自持，甚至失去理智。

【例句】 Love, hatred, and grief are emotions.

【译文】 爱、恨、悲伤都是感情。

emphasis ['emfəsis]   *n.* 强调，重点

【搭配】 lay/put/place emphasis on/upon 注重，着重于，强调

【导学】 emphasis 复数形式为 emphases（参见 analysis）。

emphasize ['emfəsaiz]   *vt.* 强调，着重

【例句】 Advertisements showed pictures of the beautiful scenery that could be enjoyed along some of the more famous western routes emphasized the romantic names of some of these trains (Empire Builder, etc).

【译文】 广告展示了在沿途能够欣赏的一些有名的西部

119

线路美丽景色的图片，而且还重点强调了一些
火车的名字（帝国建造者等）。

enable [i'neibl]　　　　　　　*vt.* 使能够，使可能

【搭配】enable sb. to do 使某人能做

endeavour [in'devə]　　　　　*vi.* 努力，尽力，尝试

【导学】近义词：attempt，aim，essay，strive，try，
effort

【例句】Apart from philosophical and legal reasons
for respecting patients' wishes, there are
several practical reasons why doctors should
endeavor to involve patients in their own
medical care decisions.

【译文】除了在道义上和法律方面要求尊重患者的愿望
之外，之所以医生努力让患者参与自己的医疗
护理决策，还有不少现实的原因。

engage [in'geidʒ]　　　　　*vt.* 使从事，使忙于；占用
（时间等）；雇用，聘用；使订婚 *vi.* 从事于，参加

【搭配】be engaged in 正忙于，从事于
be engaged to 与……订婚

enhance [in'hɑ:ns]　　　　　　　*vt.* 提高；增强

regulate ['regjuleit]　　*vt.* 管理，控制；调整，调节，
校准

【例句】 The speed of the machine may be automatically regulated to pace the packing operation by an inner microcomputer.

【译文】 机器的速度可通过内部的微型电脑自动调节得同包装速度一致。

regulation [regju'leiʃən]　*n.* 管理，控制；规章，规则

【搭配】 adopt new regulations 采取新规定
break/violate a regulation 违反规定
obey/observe regulations 遵守规定

relate [ri'leit]　*vi.* 联系，关联 *vt.* 叙述，讲述

【搭配】 be related to 与……有关系

related [ri'leitid]　*a.* 叙述的，讲述的；有关系的

relationship [ri'leiʃənʃip]　*n.* 关系，联系

relax [ri'læks]　*vt.* 使放松，使休息；缓和，放宽
vi. 放松，休息；松弛

release [ri'li:s]　*vt.* 释放，放出；发布，发行；放开，松开

【例题】 As a defense against air-pollution damage, many plants and animals _____ a substance to absorb harmful chemicals.

A. relieve   B. release

C. dismiss   D. discard   B

【译文】作为防止空气污染的屏障，许多的动植物都会
释放一种能够吸收有害化学成分的物质。

relevant [ˈrelivənt]   *a.* (to) 相关的，切题的；
                                    适当的，中肯的

【例题】 He failed to supply the facts relevant
_____ the case in question.

A. for   B. with

C. to   D. of   C

【译文】他不能够提供与该案例相关的事实依据。

reliable [riˈlaiəbl]   *a.* 可靠的

reluctant [riˈlʌktənt]   *a.* 不愿的，勉强的

【例题】 He wanted to stay at home, but at last he
agreed, very _____ though, to go to the
concert.

A. decisively   B. reluctantly

C. willingly   D. deliberately   B

【译文】他想待在家里，但是最后还是非常勉强地同意
出席音乐会。

rely [riˈlai]   *vi.* 依靠，信赖，依仗

【搭配】 rely on/upon 依靠；信赖

【例句】 The poor used to rely on government aid.

【译文】 穷人过去都依靠政府的救助。

remark [ri'mɑːk]　　　　　*n.* 评语，意见 *vt.* 说，评论
　　　　　　　　　　　　　　　　　vi. 议论，评论

【搭配】 remark on/upon 就某事发表意见

remarkable [ri'mɑːkəbl]　　　　　　　*a.* 值得注意的；
　　　　　　　　　　　　　　　　　显著的，异常的，非凡的

【例句】 A newspaper is even more remarkable for the way one reads it.

【译文】 报纸对于读者来说，阅读的方式是更值得注意的。

repetition [ˌrepi'tiʃən]　　　　　*n.* 重复，反复；背诵

【联想】 repeatedly *ad.* 重复地

【例句】 If the work of remedying of any defect or damage may affect the performance of the works, the engineer may require the repetition of any of the tests described in the contract.

【译文】 如果任何缺陷或损害的修补工作可能影响到工程运行时，工程师可要求重新进行合同中列明的任何测试。

replace [ri(ː)'pleis]　　　　　　　*vt.* 放回；替换，取代

【联想】replacement *n.* 取代，替换

【搭配】replace... with... 以……代替……

【导学】辨析 replace, substitute：replace 指取代、替换陈旧的、用坏的或遗失的东西，用法是 replace A with B（用 B 代替 A）；substitute 指用一件东西替换另一件东西，用法是 substitute B for A（用 B 代替 A）。

【例句】The new city, Brasilia, replaced Rio de Janeiro as the capital of Brazil in 1960.

【译文】1960 年，巴西利亚这座新城市取代了里约热内卢成为巴西的首都。

repopulate [ˌriːˈpɔːpjuleit]　　　*vt.* 重新入住，再生

represent [ˌriːpriˈzent]　　　*vt.* 表示，阐明，说明；描写，表现，象征；代理，代表

【搭配】represent... as 把……描述成

【例句】They elected him to represent them.

【译文】他们选他当代表。

representative [repriˈzentətiv]　　*n.* 代表，代理人
　　　　　　　　　　　　　　　　a. 典型的，有代表性的

【搭配】be representative of 有代表性的，典型的

reputation [repjuˈteiʃn]　　　*n.* 名声，声望

【搭配】have a reputation for 因……而出名

gain/acquire/establish a reputation 博得名声

reservation [ˌrezəˈveiʃən]   *n*. 预定，预订；保留

【搭配】make a reservation for 预订

【例题】When he tried to make a _____, he found that the hotel that he wanted was completely filled because of a convention.

A. complaint   B. claim

C. reservation   D. decision   C

【译文】当他想预订时，却发现他想定的酒店由于某个会议已经客满。

reserve [riˈzəːv]   *vt*. 储备；保留；预定
          n. 储备品，储备金，储备；保留地；节制，谨慎

【搭配】without reserve 毫无保留地

【例题】We'd like to _____ a table for five for dinner this evening.

A. preserve   B. sustain

C. retain   D. reserve   D

【译文】我想预订一个今晚的 5 人饭桌。

Day 11

entertain [ˌentə'tein] *vt.* 使欢乐，使娱乐；招待，款待

【联想】entertainment *n.* 娱乐，文娱节目，表演会；招待，款待，请客

enthusiasm [in'θju:ziæzəm] *n.* 热情，热心，积极性

environment [in'vaiərənmənt] *n.* 环境，四周，外界

equivalent [i'kwivələnt] *a.* 相等的；等价的，等量的
n. 同等物，等价物，对等

【例句】A mile is equivalent to about 1.6 kilometers.
【译文】1 英里大约等于 1.6 千米。

eradicate [i'rædikeit] *v.* 根除

【导学】近义词：extirpate，exterminate，annihilate；abolish，destroy

establish [is'tæbliʃ] *n.* 建立，设立，创办；确立，使确认

【联想】establishment *n.* 建立，设立，确立；建立的机构（组织）

【例句】The Minister established a commission to suggest improvements in the educational system.

【译文】部长组织了一个研究组，为改进教育制度提供建议。

estimate ['estimeit] / ['estimət]
　　　　　　　　　vt. / n. 估计，估价，评价

essence ['esns]　　　　　*n.* 本质，实质；精华，精粹

【例句】For most thinkers since the Greek philosophers, it was self-evident that there is something called human nature, something that constitutes the essence of man.

【译文】不言而喻，对于希腊哲学家及其后的大多数思想家来说，有一种叫做人性的东西，构成了人的本质。

ethical ['eθikl]　　　　*a.* （有关）道德的；伦理的；合乎道德的

evaluate [i'væljueit]　　　　　*vt.* 评价，评估

【例句】The proposal could not be evaluated because the details had not been published.

【译文】还不能评估这个建议，因为细节还没有披露。

evolve [i'vɔlv]　　　　　*v.* （使）进化，（使）演化（使）发展，（使）演变

【联想】evolution *n*. 进化，演化；发展，渐进

【例句】The developmental history of the society tells us that man has evolved from the ape.

【译文】社会发展史告诉我们：人是从类人猿进化来的。

exaggerate [igˈzædʒəreit]　　　*v*. 夸张，夸大

【例句】They exaggerated the function of the medicine.

【译文】他们夸大了这个药品的功能。

exchange [iksˈtʃeindʒ] *vt*. 交换，交流；调换，兑换
n. 交换台，交易所

【搭配】exchange A for B/substitute A for B 用 A 去换 B

excitement [ikˈsaitmənt]　　　　*n*. 刺激，兴奋

exhaust [igˈzɔːst]　　　*vt*. 用尽，耗尽，竭力；使衰竭，使精疲力竭 *n*. 排气装置，废气

【联想】exhaustion *n*. 耗尽枯竭，疲惫，筋疲力尽，竭尽

expand [iksˈpænd]　　　　*vt*. 使膨胀，详述，扩张
vi. 张开，发展

【例题】The board of the company has decided to _____ its operation to include all aspects of the clothing business.

A. extend   B. enlarge

C. expand   D. amplify   C

【译文】公司的董事会决定扩展业务范围以包含服装贸易的所有方面。

expansion [iks'pænʃən]   *n.* 扩充，开展，膨胀

expense [ik'spens]   *n.* 开销，花费；(*pl.*) 费用

【搭配】at the expense of 归……付费，以……为代价

【导学】expense 作"费用"之意时用复数形式。

experimental [iks‚peri'mentl]   *a.* 试验（上）的

explode [iks'pləud]   *v.* (使) 爆炸，爆发，破裂

【搭配】explode with anger 勃然大怒，大发脾气

      explode with laughter 哄堂大笑

【例句】It was during the morning rush hour that the bomb exploded.

【译文】爆炸是在早高峰时发生的。

exploit [iks'plɔit]   *vt.* 使用，利用；开采，开发

【例句】The Chinese government summoned people to exploit the Western China.

【译文】中国政府号召人民开发西部。

explore [iks'plɔː]   *vt.* 探险；探索，探究；勘探

【例句】Play is the most powerful way a child explores
the world and learns about himself.

【译文】玩耍是孩子探索世界和了解自身的最有力的方法。

external [eks'tə:nl] *a.* 外部的，外面的

【例句】They also need significant increases in
external financing and technical support.

【译文】他们还需要大幅度增加外部资助和技术支持。

extraordinary [iks'trɔːdnri] *a.* 非常的，特别的

extract [iks'trækt] *vt.* 取出，抽出，拔出；提取，
提炼，榨取；获得，索取；摘录，抄录
['ekstrækt] *n.* 摘录，选段；提出物，精华，汁

【例句】It is one thing to locate oil, but it is quite
another to extract and transport it to the
industrial centers.

【译文】找到石油是一回事，提炼并把石油运送到工业
中心却完全是另一回事。

facilitate [fə'siliteit] *vt.* 使便利；促进，帮助

【例句】The automatic doors in supermarkets facilitate the entry and exit of customers with
shopping carts.

【译文】超市的自动门给推购物车出入的顾客提供了便利。

facility [fəˈsiliti]　　　　　　*n.* 便利；(*pl.*) 设备，工具

【导学】作"设施"讲时，要用复数形式。

【例句】In the meeting, the government officer promised an improvement in hospitals and other health care facilities.

【译文】在会上，政府官员许诺对医院和其他医疗健康设备进行改善。

factor [ˈfæktə]　　　　　　　　　　*n.* 因素，要素

faculty [ˈfækəlti]　　　　　　*n.* 才能，本领，能力；
　　　　　　　　　　　　　　　　　全体教师；院，系

【搭配】have a faculty for sth. 有做某事的才能

【导学】做主语时，看作整体，谓语用单数形式；看作个体，谓语用复数形式。

【例句】The average number of the faculty of law in every city is forty-five.

【译文】在每个城市中平均有 45 所法学院。

fade [feid]　　　　　　　　　　　*vi.* 褪色；逐渐消失

failure [ˈfeiljə]　　　　　　*n.* 失败，不及格；失败者；
　　　　　　　　　　　　　　　　　没做到；失灵

fame [feim]   *n*. 名声，名望

【例句】 Her story shows an indifference to honors and fame can lead to great achievements.

【译文】 她的故事表明，不计较荣誉和名声也能够取得巨大的成就。

fancy ['fænsi] *n*. 想象（力）；爱好，迷恋 *a*. 别致的；异想天开的 *v*. 想象，幻想；想要，喜欢；相信；猜想

【搭配】 take a fancy to 爱好，爱上
       have a fancy for 热衷于

【导学】 后接动名词，不接动词不定式 fancy doing。

fantastic [fæn'tæstik] *a*. 空想的；奇异的，古怪的

fare [feə]   *n*. 车费，船费

【导学】 辨析 fare, fee, charge：fare 指交通费用；fee 指一种法律或组织机构规定的为某项特权而征收的固定费用，如会费、学费、入场费、报名费、手续费等，也指对职业性的服务所支付的报酬，如医生的诊费、代理人佣金、律师的胜诉金等；charge 指购买货物所付出的价钱，或获得服务所付出的费用。

【例题】 Urban crowdedness would be greatly relieved if only the charged _____ on public transport were more reasonable.

A. fees   B. fares
C. payments   D. costs

B

【译文】只有当收取公共交通费用的理由更加合理时，城市的拥挤才会得到极大的缓解。

fascinating [ˈfæsineitiŋ]   a. 迷人的，醉人的

fatal [ˈfeitl]   n. 致命的，毁灭性的

【例题】It has been proved that the chemical is <u>lethal</u> to rats but safe for cattle.
A. fatal   B. reactive
C. unique   D. vital

A

【译文】经证实，这种化学药品对于鼠类是致命的，而对家禽无害。

fate [feit]   n. 命运

【导学】辨析 fate，destiny：fate 指不可避免的命运，尤指不幸的命运；destiny 指预先注定的命运，宿命。

fatigue [fəˈtiːg]   n. 疲乏，劳累

【例句】This pill will work wonders for fatigue.

【译文】这种药片对（缓解）疲劳有神奇的效果。

faulty [ˈfɔːlti]   a. 有错误的，有缺点的

【例句】Their arguments were based on faulty reasoning.

【译文】他们的争论是基于错误的推理。

favo(u)rable ['feivərəbl]
　　　　　　　　a. 顺利的，有利的；称赞的，赞成的

【搭配】be favorable for 对某事有利
　　　　be favorable to 赞同；（对某人）有利，有益

【例句】This is the favorable weather for working outside.

【译文】这是适合户外工作的天气。

favo(u)rite ['feivərit]　　　　　*a*. 最喜爱的
　　　　　　　　　　　　　　　n. 最喜爱的人或物

【例句】Fishing is his favorite pastime on a hot summer day.

【译文】在炎热的夏日，他最喜欢的休闲方式是钓鱼。

fearful ['fiəful]　*a*. 吓人的，可怕的；害怕的，担心的

feasible ['fi:zəbl]　　　　　　　*a*. 可行的，可能的

feature ['fi:tʃə]　*n*. 面貌，容貌；特征，特色；特写

【例题】A peculiarly pointed chin is his most memorial facial _____.
　　　A. mark　　　　　B. feature
　　　C. trace　　　　　D. appearance　　　B

【译文】他那特别尖的下巴是最让人记忆犹新的面貌

特征。

federal ['fedərəl]　　　　*a.* 联邦的，联盟的，联合的

fee [fiː]　　　　*n.* 酬金；手续费；学费

feedback ['fiːdbæk]　　　　*n.* 反馈

female ['fiːmeil]　　　　*n.* 女子，雌性动物
　　　　　　　　　　　　a. 女性的，雌性的

fertile ['fəːtail]　　　　*a.* 肥沃的，富饶的；
　　　　　　　　　　　　多产的，丰富的

【例句】All the flowers are grown in the fertile soil.
【译文】所有的花都生长在肥沃的土壤里。

fertilizer ['fəːtiˌlaizə]　　　　*n.* 化肥，肥料

finance [fai'næns]　　　　*n.* 财政，金融
　　　　　　　　　　　　vt. 提供资金，接济

【联想】financial *a.* 财政的，金融的
【例句】One U. S. dollar is comparable to 131 Japanese yen according to *China Daily*'s finance news report yesterday.
【译文】据昨天《中国日报》财经新闻报道，1 美元可兑换 131 日元。

resist [ri'zist]   *vt.* 抵抗，反抗；忍住，抵制

【联想】resistance *n.* 抵抗，反抗

【例句】We must raise the Party's capacity to resist corruption.

【译文】我们必须提高党的反腐能力。

resistant [ri'zistənt]   *a.* 抵抗的，反抗的

【搭配】be resistant to 对……有抵抗力的

【例句】The researchers are already working with food companies，keen to see if their products can be made resistant to bacterial attack through alterations to the food's structure.

【译文】研究人员已经和食品公司联合起来，希望他们的产品能通过改变食品的结构来抵抗细菌的侵袭。

retail ['ri:teil]   *n.* 零售 *a.* 零售的 *v.* 零售

【搭配】sell by/at retail 零售

retain [ri'tein]   *vt.* 保持，保留

retreat [ri'tri:t]   *vi.* 撤退，退却

retrieve [ri'tri:v]   *vt.* 重新得到，取回；挽回，补救；检索

【例句】The dog was intelligent and quickly learned to retrieve the game killed by the hunter.

【译文】那狗很聪明，很快就学会了找回猎人杀死的猎物。

reveal [ri'vi:l]   *vt*. 揭示，揭露，展现；告诉，泄露

【例题】I hate people who _____ the end of a film that you haven't seen before.

A. reveal　　　　B. revise

C. rewrite　　　　D. reverse　　　A

【译文】我讨厌那些在你还没看完电影之前提前说出结局的人。

revelation [ˌrevi'leiʃən]   *n*. 揭示，透露，启示；被揭示的真相，新发现

【例句】"Spilling the beans" means confessing or making a startling revelation.

【译文】"撒了豆子"意思是坦白交代或者透露惊人的真相。

reverse [ri'vɜːs]   *v*. 颠倒，翻转，后退
　　　　　　　　　　n. /*a*. 反面（的），颠倒（的），相反（的）

【例题】Several international events in the early 1990s seem likely to _____, or at least weaken, the trends that emerged in the 1980s.

A. revolt　　　　B. revolve

C. reverse　　　　D. revive　　　C

【译文】在20世纪90年代初期的少数国际事件似乎会

扭转——至少是减弱——20 世纪 80 年代出现的
那个趋势。

rival [ˈraivəl]　　　　　　　*vt.* 竞争，与……抗衡
　　　　　　　　　　　　　　　a. 竞争的 *n.* 竞争对手

【例句】Of all the flowers in the garden few can rival
the lily.

【译文】在花园的所有花卉中，很少有花能与百合花媲
美。

romantic [rəˈmæntik]　　　　*a.* 浪漫的，传奇的；
　　　　　　　　　　　　　　　不切实际的，好幻想的

rural [ˈruər(ə)l]　　　　　　　*a.* 农村的

【例题】He pointed out that the living standard of
urban and _____ people continued to
improve.

A. remote　　　　B. municipal

C. rural　　　　　D. provincial　　　C

【译文】他指出，城市和农村地区的人们的生活水平还
在继续提高。

Day *12*

flaw [flɔː]   *n.* 缺点，裂纹，瑕疵

【例题】 The statue would be perfect but for a few small <u>defects</u> in its base.

    A. faults   B. weaknesses

    C. flaws   D. errors   C

【译文】 要不是底部部分有一些小的瑕疵，这座雕塑就很完美了。

【导学】 近义词：defect，imperfection，blemish，stain

forbid [fəˈbid]   *vt.* 禁止，不许，不准

【搭配】 forbid sb. to do sth. 禁止某人做某事

【联想】 prohibit sb. from doing sth.，prevent sb. from doing sth.，stop sb. from doing sth. 禁止某人做某事

【例句】 Waterway traffic is forbidden except on weekends.

【译文】 除了周末，水上交通工具都是禁行的。

forecast [ˈfɔːkɑːst]   *vt. / n.* 预测，预报

【导学】 辨析 forecast，predict，foretell：forecast 强调"预报"，指通过分析一些相关的信息、数

139

据来预测，这种预测是建立在科学知识或判断上的；predict 常指根据已知的事实或自然规律推断出未来的事情，可用于各种不同的场合；foretell 指凭借自己的经验或猜测能实现感觉到将来会发生的事情。

forehead [ˈfɔːhed]　　　　*n.* 额头，前额

forge [fɔːdʒ]　*n.* 锻工车间；锻炉 *v.* 锻造；伪造

formal [ˈfɔːməl]　　　　*a.* 正式的；礼仪上的；形式的

formation [fɔːˈmeiʃən] *n.* 构成；组织，形成物；地岩层

former [ˈfɔːmə]　　　　　*a.* 在前的，以前的 *n.* 前者

【搭配】the former...the latter 前者……后者

【例题】The girl was _____ a shop assistant; she is
now a manager in a large department store.
A. preliminarily　　B. presumably
C. formally　　　　D. formerly　　　D

【译文】这个女孩曾经是售货员，但现在她已经是一家大型百货公司的经理。

formula [ˈfɔːmjulə]　　　　　　*n.* 公式，程式

【搭配】formula for...　……的配方

【导学】formula 复数形式有：formulas, formulae。

formulate ['fɔːmjuleit]　　　　*vt.* 用公式表示；
　　　　　　　　　　　明确地表达；简洁陈述，阐明

fortunately ['fɔːtʃənətli]　　　　　　　*ad.* 幸亏

foundation [faun'deiʃən]　　　*n.* 成立，建立，创办；
　　　　　　　　　　基础，地基；根据；基金会

【搭配】lay a solid foundation for 为……打下坚实的
　　　　基础
【例句】The television station is supported by dona-
　　　　tion from foundations and other sources.
【译文】电视台接受来自各种基金会和其他来源的捐款
　　　　的支持。

fraction ['frækʃən] *n.* 碎片，小部分，一点儿；分数

【导学】辨析：fraction，part，portion，section，
　　　　segment，share：fraction意为"小部分，碎
　　　　片"，常表示可以略去不计的微小部分；
　　　　part纯粹为部分，并无比例内涵；portion
　　　　意为"一部分，一份"，指在某物中所占的
　　　　份额、比例；section指通过或似乎通过切割
　　　　或分离而形成的部分，如书、文章或城市的
　　　　某一部分；segment可与section换用，但更
　　　　强调某物以自然的分裂线分开的部分，或因
　　　　其结构性质而分裂的部分；share指所分享、

分担的一部分，强调共性。

fracture ['fræktʃə]　　　　　　　*n.* 破裂，骨折

　　　　　　　　　　　　　　　　v. (使) 破碎，(使) 破裂

fragile ['frædʒail]　　　*a.* 脆的；虚弱的；易碎的

【例句】 Dispossessed peasants slash and burn their way into the rain forests of Latin America，and hungry nomads turn their herds out onto fragile African grassland，reducing it to desert.

【译文】 被剥夺得一无所有的农民在拉丁美洲的热带雨林中砍伐和焚烧，而饥饿的游牧民族把他们的家畜赶进了脆弱的非洲草原，使其退化成沙漠。

fragment ['frægmənt]　　　*n.* 碎片，小部分，片断

frustrate [frʌs'treit] *vt.* 破坏，阻挠；使失败，使泄气

【例句】 After three hours' frustrating delay, the train at last arrived.

【译文】 经过 3 个小时令人心烦的耽搁后，火车终于到达了目的地。

fundamental [ˌfʌndə'mentl]　　　*a.* 基础的，根本的，重要的 *n.* (*pl.*) 基本原则，基本原理

【搭配】 be fundamental to 对……必不可少

【联想】 be essential to, be vital to 对……至关重要

【例句】 These experts say that we must understand the fundamental relation between ourselves and wild animals.

【译文】 这些专家说，我们必须明白我们自己和野生动物之间的重要关系。

fungal ['fʌŋgl]   *a.* 真菌的；真菌引起的

gap [gæp]   *n.* 缺口，间隔；隔阂，差距

【搭配】 bridge the gap between 弥合（……之间的）差别；消除隔阂；bridge/fill/stop/close a gap 弥补不足；填补空白

【例句】 There are wide gaps in my knowledge of history.

【译文】 我很缺乏历史知识。

gas [gæs]   *n.* 煤气；气体；汽油

【联想】 gasoline *n.* 汽油

gastric ['gæstrik]   *a.* 胃的；胃部的

gear [giə]   *n.* 齿轮，传动装置；用具，装备
                                          v. 开动，连接

【搭配】 gear up （使）准备好，（使）做好安排
        gear... to 使……适合

【例句】 Education should be geared to children's needs.

【译文】教育应适合孩子们的需要。

gene [dʒiːn]   *n.* 基因

【例句】 Most of us inherit half our gene from our mothers and half from our fathers.

【译文】 我们大多数人继承一半母亲的基因，一半父亲的基因。

generalize ['dʒenərəlaiz]   *v.* 概括，归纳，推断

【联想】 generalized 是形容词，意为"广泛的，普及的"。

【例句】 In the emic approach the researchers might choose to focus only on middle-class white families without regard for whether the information obtained in the study can be generalized or is appropriate for ethnic minority groups.

【译文】 使用着位法，研究者可能只注意到那些白人中产阶级家庭，全然不考虑研究中所获得信息是否有普遍性或者对少数民族群体是否合适。

genetic [dʒi'netik]   *a.* 遗传的，起源的

【例句】 The human population contains a great variety of genetic variation, but drugs are tested on just a few thousand people.

【译文】 人类具有各种各样的遗传变异，可是药品的试

验只能在数千人中进行。

generally [ˈdʒenərəli]   *ad.* 一般，通常

generate [ˈdʒenəreit]   *vt.* 产生，发生；引起，导致
【例句】When coal burns, it generates heat.
【译文】煤燃烧时，产生热量。

generator [ˈdʒenəreitə]   *n.* 发电机，发生器

generous [ˈdʒenərəs]   *a.* 慷慨的，大方的；
                                      丰盛的，丰富的；宽厚的

【搭配】be generous to sb. 对某人宽大；be generous with sth. 用某物大方

【例题】He made such a _____ contribution to the university that they are naming one of the new buildings after him.
    A. genuine   B. minimum
    C. modest   D. generous   D

【译文】他给大学如此慷慨的捐助，所以他们将以他的名字给其中一座新楼命名。

genius [ˈdʒiːnjəs]   *n.* 天才

【联想】have a faculty for，have a gift for，have a talent for，have a capacity for 具有……的才能/天赋

【导学】辨析 genius, gift, talent：genius 指天赋，超常的智力和创造力，具有这种天赋的人极为罕见；gift 指天资，才能，通常被认为是生来就有的某一方面突出的才能；talent 指生来即有的天分或能力，通常需要加以培养和发展。

【例句】I was going to be a complete engineer, technical genius and sensitive humanist all in one.

【译文】我想做一个真正意义上的工程师，技术上的天才和敏感的人文学者集于一身的工程师。

genuine [ˈdʒenjuin]　　　　　*a.* 真实的，真正的；真心的，真诚的

【例句】The questions usually grow out of their genuine interest or curiosity.

【译文】问题通常来自他们真正的兴趣或好奇心。

global [ˈgləubəl]　　　　　*a.* 地球的，全球的；全局的

globe [gləub]　　　　　*n.* 地球；地球仪，球体

【例句】We believe it is a reasonable real-world test of good manners around the globe.

【译文】我们相信这是一个世界范围内的、合理的、现实的关于礼貌的测试。

grace [greis]   *n.* 优美，雅致；(*pl.*) 风度，魅力

【联想】graceful *a.* 优美的，文雅的

gradual ['grædjuəl]   *a.* 逐渐的，逐步的

graduate ['grædjuət]   *n.* 毕业生；研究生
          ['grædʒueit]   *vi.* 毕业

【联想】undergraduate *n.* 大学本科生；postgraduate *n.* 研究生；bachelor *n.* 学士；master *n.* 硕士；doctor，Ph. D *n.* 博士

【例句】23-year-old Eric graduated from college last year.

【译文】23 岁的埃里克去年从大学毕业了。

grant [grɑːnt]   *n.* 拨款；准许 *v.* 准予，授予，同意

【搭配】take... for granted 认为……理所当然

【例句】The government gave us a grant to build another classroom.

【译文】政府给了我们一笔补助，用来盖另外一间教室。

gratitude ['grætitjuːd]   *n.* 感激，感谢

【例题】I would like to express my _____ to you all for supporting me this summer as a visiting scholar in your department.

    A. satisfaction   B. gratitude

147

C. pleasure   D. sincerity   B

【译文】 我想要向你们表示感激，因为在今年夏天我作为访问学者对贵系进行访问期间你们给我提供了支持。

guarantee [ˌɡærənˈtiː]   *n.* 保证，保证书
                              vt. 保证，担保

【导学】 辨析 guarantee, pledge, warranty：guarantee 意为"担保，保证，抵押品"，指对事物的品质或人的行为提出担保，常暗示双方有法律上或其他方式的默契，保证补偿不履行所造成的损失；pledge 意为"保证，誓约，抵押品"，为普通用语，可泛指保证忠实于某种原则或接受并尽忠某一职责的庄严保证或诺言，但这都是以跟人的信誉作保证的承诺；warranty 指"（商品的）保证书，保单，保证"，如修理或退还残缺货物等。

【例句】 Nuclear power, with all its inherent problems, is still the only option to guarantee enough energy in the future.

【译文】 虽然核动力还存在它固有的问题，但它仍然是将来有足够能源的唯一保证。

guidance [ˈɡaidəns]   *n.* 引导，指导

【搭配】 under the guidance of 在……引导之下

pace [peis]　　　　　　　*n.* (一) 步，步子；步速，速度

【搭配】keep/lead pace with（与……）并驾齐驱，保
　　　　持一致；set the pace 起带头作用

【导学】辨析 pace，rate，speed，velocity：pace 意
　　　　为"步速，速度，进度"，也指运动的速率，
　　　　多指走路的人、跑步的人或小跑的马匹的行
　　　　速，用于比喻时指各种活动、生产效率等发
　　　　展的速度；rate 意为"速率，比率"，用与其
　　　　他事物的关系来衡量速度、价值、成本等，
　　　　作速度讲时强调单位时间内的速度；speed
　　　　意为"速率，速度"，指任何事物持续运动
　　　　时的速度，尤指车辆等无生命事物的运动速
　　　　度；velocity 意为"速度"，技术用语，指物
　　　　体沿着特定方向运动时的速率。

package ['pækidʒ]　　　　　　*n.* 包装，包裹，箱；
　　　　　　　　　　　　　　　　　一揽子交易（或计划、建议等）

【搭配】a package deal/offer 一揽子交易

pact [pækt]　　　　　　　　*n.* 协定，条约；契约

【例句】The trade pact between those two countries
　　　　come to an end.

【译文】那两个国家的通商协定宣告结束。

painful ['peinful]　　　　　　　*a.* 痛苦的，疼痛的；
　　　　　　　　　　　　　　　困难，令人不快的

palm [pɑːm]　　　　　　　　　　　*n.* 手掌

【搭配】palm off 用欺骗手段把……卖掉；grease/oil
one's palm 贿赂某人；have an itching palm
贪财；in the palm of one's hand 在某人的完
全控制之下；know sth. like the palm of
one's hand 对某事了如指掌

pandemic [pæn'demɪk]　　　*n.* (全国或全球性)
　　　　　　　　　　　　　　流行病；大流行病
　　　　　　　　a. (疾病) 大流行的；普遍的，全世界的

【例句】Experts say that global cooperation is essential for pandemic control.

【译文】专家表示，全球合作对疫情控制至关重要。

panel ['pænl] *n.* 专门小组；面板，控制板，仪表盘

panic ['pænɪk]　　*n.* 惊慌，恐慌 *a.* 恐慌的，惊慌的

paradox ['pærədɔks]　　　　　*n.* 似乎矛盾而 (可能)
　　　　　正确的说法；自相矛盾的人 (或事情)

【例句】We work to make money，but it's a paradox
that people who work hard and long often

don't make the most money.

【译文】 我们工作是为了挣钱，但矛盾的是，那些工作辛苦、时间又长的人经常并不是挣钱最多的人。

paralyze ['pærəlaiz]   *vt.* 使瘫痪，使麻痹；使丧失作用；使惊愕，使呆若木鸡

【例句】 In May, Julie Nimmus, president of Schutt Sports in Illinois, successfully fought a lawsuit involving a football player who was paralyzed in a game while wearing a Schutt helmet.

【译文】 5 月，伊利诺伊州舒特体育用品公司的总裁朱利·尼姆斯打赢了一场官司，原告是一名橄榄球队员，他戴着舒特公司的头盔在一场比赛中受伤瘫痪。

parental [pə'rentl]   *a.* 父母的，父（母）亲的

partial ['pɑːʃəl]   *a.* 部分的，局部的；偏爱的，不公平的

【例句】 The research project was only a partial success.

【译文】 那个研究课题只取得了部分成功。

participate [pɑː'tisipeit]   *vi.* 参与，参加

【搭配】 participate in 参加，参与

【例句】 Americans want to participate in all kinds of

activities.

【译文】美国人想参加各种各样的活动。

particle [ˈpɑːtikl]   *n.* 粒子，微粒

particularly [pəˈtikjuləli]   *ad.* 特别地，尤其地

passion [ˈpæʃən]   *n.* 激情，热情；酷爱

【搭配】have a passion for 喜爱
        be passionate for 对……热衷，对……热爱

【例句】His skill as a player doesn't quite match his passion for the game.

【译文】他的水平与他对这项游戏的酷爱程度不太相配。

patch [pætʃ]   *n.* 小片，小块，补丁 *vt.* 补，修补

【搭配】patch up 解决（争吵、麻烦）等；修补，草草修理

patent [ˈpætənt]   *n.* 专利权，专利品
                                           vt. 取得……的专利权，请准专利
        [ˈpeitnt]   *a.* 特许的，专利的

【例句】Communications technology is generally exported from the U. S. , Europe, or Japan; the patents skills and ability to manufacture remain in the hands of a few industrialized countries.

【译文】通信技术一般是由美国、欧洲和日本出口的，专利技术技能和制造能力掌握在一些工业化国家手中。

pathogen [ˈpæθədʒɛn]　　　　　　　　　*n*. 病原体

pathology [pəˈθɒlədʒi]　　　　　　　　*n*. 病理学

patience [ˈpeiʃəns]　　　　　　　　*n*. 忍耐，耐心

【搭配】run out one's patience 失去耐心
　　　　with patience 耐心地
　　　　out of patience with 对……失去耐心

payment [ˈpeimənt]　　　　　　　　*n*. 支付，付款

【搭配】in payment for 以偿付，以回报

peculiar [piˈkju:ljə]　　　*a*. 特殊的，独特的；古怪的

【搭配】be peculiar to 是……所特有的
【联想】specific to 特有的；proper to 特有的，固有的

pediatrics [ˌpi:diˈætriks]　　　　　　　　*n*. 儿科

penetrate [ˈpenitreit]　　　　*v*. 穿透，渗入，看穿

【搭配】penetrate through/into 穿过，渗透

performance [pəˈfɔ:məns]　　　　*n*. 表演，演出；
　　　　　　　　　　执行，完成；工作情况，表现情况

153

permanent [ˈpəːmənənt]　　　　　*a.* 永久的，持久的

【导学】 permanent，perpetual，eternal：permanent
指永久不变的，与暂时相对；perpetual 指动
作无休止进行或状态无休止继续；eternal 表
示无始无终的，永恒的。

personality [ˌpəːsəˈnæliti]　　　　*n.* 人格，个性

【例句】 Personality in Americans is further complicated by successive waves of immigration from
various countries.

【译文】 由于一波接一波外国移民的移入，美国人的性
格更复杂了。

personnel [ˌpəːsəˈnel]　　　　　*n.* 全体人员，
全体职员；人事部门

【导学】 personnel 作全体员工讲时，是集合名词，所
以做主语时谓语用复数。

Day *13*

handful [ˈhændful] 　　　　　　　　 *n*. 一把，一小撮

handle [ˈhændl] 　　　　　　 *n*. 柄，把手，拉手
　　　　　 vt. 触，摸，抚弄；操纵；处理，应付

handy [ˈhændi] 　　　　 *a*. 手边的，近处的；方便的
【联想】handiness *n*. 可用，方便

harass [ˈhærəs] 　　　　 *vt*. 使疲乏，困扰，反复袭击
【联想】barassment *n*. 骚扰，侵袭；烦恼
【例题】A number of black youths have complained of
　　　　being _____ by the police.
　　　　A. harassed　　　B. distracted
　　　　C. sentenced　　　D. released 　　　A
【译文】许多黑人青年抱怨被警察骚扰。

harm [hɑːm] 　　　　　　 *n*. / *vt*. 损害，伤害，危害
【联想】harmful *a*. 有害的；伤害的
【搭配】come to no harm 未受到伤害
　　　　do harm to 损害，对……有害
【例句】Breathing in other people's cigarette smoke

155

can do real harm to your lungs.

【译文】吸入二手烟会对你的肺有损害。

harmony ['hɑːməni]   *n*. 和谐，和睦，融洽

【联想】harmoniou *a*. 和谐的

【搭配】in harmony with（与……）协调一致；（与……）和睦相处

【例句】Design criteria include harmony of colour, texture, lighting, scale, and proportion.

【译文】设计的准则包括色彩、材质、照明、比例的协调。

hatred ['heitrid]   *n*. 憎恶，憎恨，怨恨

hazard ['hæzəd]   *n*. 危险，危害，公害

【联想】hazardous *a*. 危险的；冒险的；危害的

【搭配】at hazard, in danger 在危险中；at all hazards 不顾一切危险；on the hazard 受到威胁；take a hazard to do 冒险做；run the hazard / risk of doing 冒险

headline ['hedlain]   *n*. 大标题

【导学】辨析 heading, headline：heading 指文章定的标题、题目，也指谈话的论题、话题；headline 指报刊的大字标题、页头题目等。

heal [hiːl]   *v.* 治愈，愈合

【搭配】heal sb. of sth. 治愈某人的病

healthcare [ˈhelθkeə]   *n.* 医疗保健，健康护理

hernia [ˈhəːniə]   *n.* 疝

hippocampus [ˌhipəˈkæmpəs]   *n.* 海马体
        (大脑中被认为是感情和记忆中心的部分)

historical [hisˈtɔrikəl]   *a.* 历史的，有关历史的

【导学】辨析 historical，historic：historical 指历史上
       存在或发生过的；historic 指历史上有名的，
       有历史意义的。

host [həust]   *n.* 主人，旅店老板；节目主持人

【导学】辨析 host，master：host 与 guest（客人）相
       对，即 host 招待的是 guests；master 与
       servant（仆人）相对，即 master 指使的是
       servant。

hospitality [ˌhɔspiˈtæliti]   *n.* (对客人的)
                      友好款待，好客

【导学】以-able 结尾的形容词变成名词时，往往只需
       将-able 变为-ability，例如：able（能……的，
       有才能的）→ability（能力，才干），capable

（有能力的，能干的）→ capability（能力，
性能，容量），changeable（可改变的）→
changeability（可变性，易变性），但是请注
意 hospitable（好客的，招待周到的）→
hospitality（好客，殷勤）。

【例句】 Thank you so much for your generous hospitality.
【译文】 非常感谢您的盛情款待。

humane [hjuːˈmein]　　　　 a. 善良的；仁慈的；人道的

humanity [hjuːˈmænəti]　　　　 n. 人性；人类；人道；
（统称）人；仁慈；人文学科

ideal [aiˈdiəl]　　 a. 理想的，称心如意的；唯心论的
n. 理想

identical [aiˈdentikəl]　　　 a. 相同的；同一的

【搭配】 be identical with/to 和……完全相同
be identical in 在……方面相同

【导学】 辨析 be similar to, be the same as, be
identical with/to：be similar to 和……相似；
be the same as 和……相同；be identical
with/to 和……完全相同。

【例题】 The jobs of wildlife technicians and biologists
seemed _____ to him, but one day he
discovered their difference.

A. identical   B. vertical

C. parallel   D. specific   A

【译文】 在他看来，似乎野生动植物技术员和生物学家的工作是一样的，但是有一天他发现了他们之间的区别。

identify [aɪˈdentɪfaɪ]   *vt.* 认出，鉴定；等同，打成一片

【搭配】 identify oneself with... 参加到……中去；identify...with 认为……等同于

【导学】 辨析 identify，recognize：identify 指通过某些内在的东西辨认出某人某物；recognize 指认出曾经见过或原来认识的人或物，强调通过外表认出。

【例句】 Verification of the product can be carried out in the process in order to identify variation.

【译文】 产品的验证可在运行过程中进行，以便识别变化。

identification [aɪˌdentɪfɪˈkeɪʃən]   *n.* 辨认，视为同一；证明，鉴定

【搭配】 identification card = identity card 身份证

【例句】 He used a letter of introduction as identification.

【译文】 他用一封介绍信作为身份的证明。

identity [aɪˈdentɪtɪ]   *n.* 身份；个性，特征

【例题】The police are trying to find out the _____ of the woman killed in the traffic accident.

A. evidence   B. recognition

C. status   D. identity   D

【译文】警方正在设法查清那名在交通事故中受害的女性的身份。

ignorance ['ignərəns]   *n.* 无知，愚昧

【例句】Ignorance of the law is no excuse.

【译文】不懂法律不能成为借口。

ignorant ['ignərənt]   *a.* 无知的，愚昧的；不知道的

【搭配】be ignorant of/that... 不知道，不了解

【例句】A tiny insect, trying to shake a mighty tree, is ludicrously ignorant of its own weakness.

【译文】蚍蜉撼大树，可笑不自量。

illegal [i'li:gəl]   *a.* 不合法的，非法的

【例句】Selling cigars without a license is illegal.

【译文】无执照销售雪茄烟是违法的。

illustrate ['iləstreit]   *vt.* 举例说明，图解

【例题】The following account by the author _____ the difference between European and American reactions.

A. illustrates   B. acquires

C. demands　　　D. deletes 　　A

【译文】作者做出的下列解释说明了欧洲人和美国人在反应方面的区别。

image ['imidʒ] 　　*n.* 像；肖像，形象；影像，图像

【联想】imagination *n.* 想象，想象力；空想，幻想

imaginable [i'mædʒinəbl] 　　*a.* 可想象到的，可能的

imaginary [i'mædʒinəri] *a.* 想象的，虚构的，假想的

【例题】All the characters in the play are _____.
　　A. imaginable　　B. imaginary
　　C. imaginative　　D. imagining 　　B

【译文】剧中所有的人物都是虚构的。

imaginative [i'mædʒinətiv] *a.* 富有想象力的，爱想象的

【导学】注意 imaginative 和 imaginary 虽然都是形容词，但它们的意思还是有区别的，imaginative 常用来形容某人富有想象力，喜欢想象，而 imaginary 多用来形容某事物或某故事是假想的，虚构的，例如：He is an imaginative writer. 他是一个富有想象力的作家。He told a story about an imaginary land. 他讲了一个关于虚构的地方的故事。

【例句】She is a very imaginative student. She's always talking about traveling to outer space.

【译文】她是一个富有想象力的学生，总是谈论关于遨游外太空的事情。

immediately [i'miːdjətli]　　　*ad*. 立即，马上，直接

pharmaceutical [ˌfɑːmə'suːtikl]　*a*. 制药的，配药的

pharmacy ['fɑːməsi]　　　*n*. 药房，药剂学，配药业，制药业

phase [feiz]　　　　　　　　*n*. 阶段，时期；月相

【搭配】phase in 逐步采用；phase out 逐步停止；out of phase with 与……不协调；in phase with 与……协调

phenomenon [fi'nɔminən]　　　　　*n*. 现象

【导学】phenomenon 复数形式为 phenomena。

phrase [freiz]　　　　　*n*. 短语，词组，习语

physical ['fizikəl]　　　*a*. 物质的，有形的；身体的；自然科学的，物理的

【搭配】physical education 体育；physical strength 体力；physical constitution 体格

【例句】When a danger is psychological rather than physical，fear can force you to take self-protective measures.

【译文】 当出现心理危险而非身体危险时，恐惧会迫使你采取自我保护措施。

physician [fi'ziʃən]   *n.* 内科医生

【联想】 doctor 医生（一般用语）；practitioner *n.* （医生、律师等）开业者；surgeon *n.* 外科医生；dentist *n.* 牙医

physicist ['fizisist]   *n.* 物理学家

plague [pleig]   *n.* 瘟疫；麻烦，苦恼，灾祸
                                                      vt. 折磨，使苦恼

pleased [pli:zd]   *a.* 高兴的，满足的

politician [pɔli'tiʃən]   *n.* 政治家，政客

【联想】 statesman *n.* 政治家（含褒义）

politics ['pɔlitiks]   *n.* 政治；政见，政纲

pollute [pə'lu:t]   *vt.* 污染，玷污

【联想】 pollution *n.* 污染；pollutant *n.* 污染物质

populate ['pɔpjuleit]   *v.* 使人民居住，移民

【联想】 population *n.* 人口

portable ['pɔːtəbl]   *a.* 轻便的，手提（式）的

【例句】The documents have been typed into a portable computer.

【译文】文件已经被输入到一台便携式电脑里了。

portrait ['pɔːtrit]   *n.* 肖像，画像

potential [pə'tenʃ(ə)l]   *a.* 潜在的，可能的
                                        n. 潜力，潜能

【例句】It's much to be regretted that he died so young, his potential unfulfilled.

【译文】他才华未展，英年早逝，十分令人惋惜。

practicable ['præktikəbl]   *a.* 能实行的，
                                        行得通的，可以实行的

【联想】practically *ad.* 实际上；几乎

practitioner [præk'tiʃənə]   *n.* 开业医生；律师

precaution [pri'kɔːʃn]   *n.* 预防，留心，警戒
                                        vt. 预告，警告

【例句】Our first priority is to take every precaution to protect our citizens at home and around the world from further attacks.

【译文】我们首要任务是采取一切预防措施，以保证我们的公民不论是在家还是在世界上的其他地方

都不再受到袭击。

pregnant ['pregnənt]　　　　　　　　*a.* 怀孕的

【联想】pregnancy *n.* 怀孕，怀孕期

premature [ˌpremə'tjuə]　　　　　*a.* 未成熟的，早熟的

preliminary [pri'liminəri]　　　　*a.* 预备的，初步的

prenatal [ˌpri:'neitl]　　　　　　　*a.* 孕期的

preparation [ˌprepə'reiʃən]　　　*n.* 准备，预备；
　　　　　　　　　　　　　　　　　　 制备品，制剂

【搭配】make preparations for 为……做准备；in
　　　　preparation 在准备中；in preparation for 作
　　　　为……的准备

prescribe [pris'kraib] *vt.* 开处方，开药；规定，指示

【搭配】prescribe for 为……开处方

【例句】The doctor prescribed his patient a receipt.

【译文】医生给病人开了一张药方。

presence ['prezns]　　　　　　*n.* 出席，在场；存在

【搭配】in the presence of sb. 当着某人的面，有某人
　　　　在场；presence of mind 镇定自若

presentation [ˌprezen'teiʃən] *n.* 介绍，陈述；表现形式

presumably [prɪˈzjuːməbli]　　　　*ad.* 推测上，大概

prevail [prɪˈveɪl]　　*vi.* 取胜，占优势；流行，盛行

【搭配】prevail over/against 战胜，压倒；prevail in/
　　　　among 流行，普遍存在；prevail on/upon sb.
　　　　to do sth. 劝说某人做某事

【例题】Nothing is so uncertain as the fashion market
　　　　where　one　style　_____　over　another
　　　　before being replaced.
　　　　A. dominates　　　B. manipulates
　　　　C. overwhelms　　 D. prevails　　　　　D

【译文】没有什么比时尚界更不确定的了，一种时装样
　　　　式在被取代前，和其他样式相比都占优势地位。

prevalent [ˈprevələnt]　　　　　　*n.* 流行的，普遍的

【导学】近义词：widespread，accepted，common，
　　　　prevailing

primary [ˈpraɪməri]　　*a.* 首要的，主要的，基本的；
　　　　　　　　　　　　　　　　　　最初的，初级的

probable [ˈprɒbəbl] *a.* 有希望的，可能的；也许，大概

procedure [prəˈsiːdʒə]　　　　　　　　　　　　*n.* 程序

proceed [prə'siːd]　　　　　　　　*vi.* 继续进行

【搭配】 proceed to do sth. 继续做（另一件事）
　　　　 proceed with sth. 继续进行

【例句】 Once your PIN has been reset, you may proceed to create a new PIN.

【译文】 一旦您的 PIN 被重新设置，您就可以继续创建新的 PIN。

profession [prə'feʃən]　　　　　*n.* 职业，自由职业

【搭配】 by profession 在职业上，就职业而言

professional [prə'feʃənl]　　　　*a.* 职业的，专门的
　　　　　　　　　　　　　　　　　　n. 专业人员

【例句】 He has just turned professional.

【译文】 他刚成为专业人士。

Day *14*

immigrant ['imigrənt]　　　*n.* 移民，侨民 *a.* 移民的

【导学】辨析 immigrant，emigrant：immigrant 指的
是来自国外的移民，指为了永久居住而从别
国到居住国的人；emigrant 指的是离开国家
或地区到别国永久居住的人。

impact ['impækt]　　　*n.* 影响，作用；冲击，碰撞

【搭配】have an impact on sth. 对……的影响

【例题】Professor Taylor's talk has indicated that science
has a very strong _____ on the everyday life
of nonscientists as well as scientists.

　　　A. motivation　　　B. perspective

　　　C. impression　　　D. impact　　　D

【译文】泰勒教授指出，科学对科学家和普通人的日常
生活都会产生强烈的影响。

impair [im'pɛə]　　　*v.* 损害，损伤，削弱

【导学】近义词：spoil，injure，hurt，damage，destroy；
diminish，undermine，reduce，weaken

【例题】Memory can be both enhanced and <u>impaired</u>
by use of drugs.

A. inhibited   B. injured

C. induced   D. intervened   B

【译文】使用药物可以提高也可以削弱记忆。

imperative [im'perətiv] *a.* 必要的，紧急的，极重的；命令的 *n.* 必要的事，必须完成的事；祈使语气

【例句】Military orders are imperative and cannot be disobeyed.

【译文】军令是强制性的，必须遵守。

impatient [im'peiʃənt]   *a.* 不耐烦的，急躁的

【搭配】be impatient of 对……不耐烦，不能忍受

be impatient for/to do 急切

implicate ['implikeit] *vt.* 牵连；牵涉，涉及（某人）；表明（或意指）……是起因

【例句】He tried to avoid saying anything that would implicate him further.

【译文】他尽力避免说出任何会进一步牵连他的事情。

inadequate [in'ædikwət]   *a.* 不充分的；不足的；不够的；不胜任的

【例句】The supplies of food are inadequate to meet the needs.

【译文】食物供给还不能充分满足需求。

incidence ['insidəns] *n.* 发生（率）

【例句】 At present, it is not possible to confirm or to refute the suggestion that there is a causal relationship between the amount of fat we eat and the incidence of heart attacks.

【译文】 目前我们很难决定应该赞成还是反驳这种观点，即脂肪的摄入量和心脏发病率之间存在着因果关系。

incidentally [insi'dentəli] *ad.* 附带提及地，顺便地

【导学】 有些副词用来表示评价一件事，或说明一种状态，可以单独放在句首，除 incidentally 以外，常见的还有：fortunately 幸运的是，unfortunately 不幸地，luckily 幸运地，generally（或 generally speaking）一般说来。

【例句】 I must go now. Incidentally, if you want that book I'll bring it next time.

【译文】 我现在该走了。顺便提一句，如果你要那本书，我下次带来。

incident ['insidənt] *n.* 事件，政治事件，事变

【例题】 Have you a funny _____ or unusual experience that you would like to share?

　　A. amusement　　B. incident

　　C. accident　　D. section　　　B

【译文】你有什么有趣的或者非凡的经历来分享吗？

incline [inˈklain]　　　　v. 使倾向，使倾斜，使偏向
　　　　　　　　　　　　　　n. 斜坡，斜面

【搭配】incline to/towards sth. 有……的倾向；be inclined to do sth. 想做某事，有……的趋势

incorporate [inˈkɔːpəreit]　　　　vt. 结合，合并，使加入，收编 vi. 合并，混合

【例句】We will incorporate your suggestion in the new plan.

【译文】我们将把你的建议纳入新计划。

increasingly [inˈkriːsiŋli]　　　ad. 日益地，越来越多地

【例题】The international situation has been growing _____ difficult for the last few years.
　　　A. invariably　　　B. presumably
　　　C. increasingly　　D. dominantly　　C

【译文】最近几年国际形势越来越严峻。

indicate [ˈindikeit]　　　　vt. 指示，表示；暗示

【联想】indication n. 指示，表示；暗示

indicator [ˈindikeitə]　　　n. 指示器，指示剂；
　　　　　　　　　　　　　　　[计算机] 指示符

【例题】If exercise is a bodily maintenance activity

and an <u>index</u> of physiological age, the lack of
sufficient exercise may either cause or hasten
aging.

A. instance   B. indicator

C. appearance   D. option   B

【译文】 如果锻炼能够维持身体机能同时也可成为生理
年龄指标，那么缺乏足够的锻炼可能会造成衰
老，也可能会加速衰老。

individual [ˌindiˈvidjuəl] *a.* 个别的，单独的；独特的
                        n. 个人，个体

【导学】 辨析 individual, personal, private：individu-
al 意为"独立于他人的，各个的，个别的"，
与 general（普遍的）和 collective（集体的）
相对；personal 意思是"个人的，亲自的"；
private 意为"私人的，秘密的"，与 public
（公共的，共有的）相对。

【例句】 The other reasons to oppose the death penalty
are largely a matter of individual conscience
and belief.

【译文】 另外一个反对死刑的原因主要是个人良知和信
仰的问题。

industrial [inˈdʌstriəl]   *a.* 工业的；产业的

【导学】 辨析 industrial, industrious：industrial 意为

"工业的，产业的"；industrious 意为"勤劳的，勤奋的"。

inevitable [in'evitəbl]　　　　*a.* 不可避免的，必然的

【例句】It is inevitable that some changes will take place.

【译文】有些变化将要发生，不可避免。

infant ['infənt]　　　　　　　　*n.* 婴儿，幼儿

Inflame [in'fleim]　　*vt.* 使（局势）恶化；激起……的强烈感情

inflation [in'fleiʃən]　　　　　*n.* 通货膨胀

influence ['influəns]　　　　　*n.* 势力，权势
　　　　　　　　　　　　　　　vt. /n. 影响，感化

【搭配】have influence on/upon 影响

【联想】influential *a.* 有影响的，有势力的

【例句】It also has some negative influence.

【译文】这也有一些负面影响。

infrastracture ['infrəstrʌktʃə(r)]
　　　　　　　　　　　　　　n. 基础设施，基础建设

inform [in'fɔːm] *vt.* 通知，告诉，报告；告发，告密

【搭配】inform sb. of sth. 把某事告知某人

inform against/on sb. 告发，检举某人

【导学】辨析 inform, notify：inform 意为"告诉，通知"，强调直接把任何种类的事实或知识告诉或传递给某人；notify 意为"通知"，指用官方公告或正式通知书将所应该或需要知道的事告诉某人，含有情况紧急，需要立刻采取行动或及早答复的意思。

initial [iˈniʃəl]   *a.* 最初的，开头的 *n.* 首字母

【导学】辨析 initial, original, primary, primitive：initial 意为"最初的，开始的"，强调处于事物的起始阶段的，开头的，也可指位于开头地方的；original 意为"最早的，最先的"，强调处于事物的起始阶段的，按顺序应是首位的，也可指原始的、原件的，即非仿造的东西；primar 指在时间、顺序或发展上领先的（第一的、基本的、主要的）；primitive 指处于人类生命或事物发展的早期阶段的、原始的。

initiate [iˈniʃieit]   *vt.* 开始，创始，发动；
启蒙，使入门；引入，正式介绍

【搭配】be initiated into 正式加入；initiate sb. into sth. 准许或介绍某人加入某团体，把某事传

授给某人

【例句】We should initiate a new social custom.

【译文】我们要开创社会新风尚。

initiative [iˈniʃiətiv]   *n.* 创始，首创精神；
                                   决断的能力；主动性 *a.* 起始的，初步的

【例题】Two decade ago a woman who shook hands
with men on her own _____ was usually
viewed as too forward.

    A. endeavor   B. initiative

    C. motivation   D. preference   **B**

【译文】20 年前，主动和男性握手的女性通常被认为是
非常前卫的人。

innocent [ˈinəsnt]   *a.* 无罪的，清白的；
                               无害的；天真的，单纯的

【搭配】be innocent of 无意识的，无……罪的

【联想】be guilty of 有……罪

innovation [ˌinəuˈveiʃən]   *n.* 创新，改革

【例句】Given this optimistic approach to technologi-
cal innovation，the American worker took
readily to that special kind of nonverbal
thinking required in mechanical technology.

【译文】有了这种对技术革新的乐观态度，美国工人

很快便习惯了机械技术所需要的非语言的思维方式。

intact [in'tækt]   *a*. 未经触动的，原封不动的，完整无损的

intake ['inteik]   *n*. 摄入；（食物、饮料等的）摄取量，吸入量；（一定时期内）纳入的人数；吸收

insomnia [in'sɔmniə]   *n*. 失眠症

inspect [in'spekt]   *vt*. 检查，调查，视察

【例题】 All factories and mines are _____ by government officials.
　　　A. examined　　　 B. surveyed
　　　C. inspected　　　 D. investigated　　　C
【译文】 所有工矿企业都要接受政府官员的视察。

install [in'stɔ:l]   *vt*. 安装，设置
【联想】 installation *n*. 安装，设置

installment [in'stɔ:lmənt]   *n*. 分期付款；（连载的）一部分，一期

【例句】 We pay for our holidays in installment of $ 50 a month.
【译文】 我们以每月50美元分期付款的方式度假。

instance [ˈinstəns] 　　　　　　　*n.* 例证，实例

【搭配】for instance 举例说，比如

instant [ˈinstənt] *n.* 瞬间，时刻 *a.* 立即的，立刻的；紧急的，迫切的；（食品）速溶的，方便的

【搭配】on the instant 立即；the instant（that）一······就（引导时间状语从句）

【例题】You see the lightening _____ it happens, but you hear the thunder later.

A. the instant　　 B. for an instant
C. on the instant　 D. in an instant 　　Ⓐ

【译文】你可以在闪电发生的瞬间立刻看见它，但要稍后才能听到雷声。

insurance [inˈʃuərəns] 　　　　　　*n.* 保险，保险费

【例题】After the robbery, the shop installed a sophisticated alarm system as an insurance _____ further losses.

A. for　　　　 B. from
C. against　　 D. towards 　　Ⓒ

【译文】抢劫发生以后，商店装了一套精密复杂的警报系统，以防止进一步的损失。

insure [inˈʃuə] 　　　　　*vi.* 保险，替······保险；保证

【搭配】insure sb./sth. against 给某人或某物保险以防

【联想】assure sb. of sth. /that 使某人确信；convince sb. of sth., ensure sth. 确保某事；make sure that 保证

【例句】It is advisable to insure your life against accident.

【译文】最好参加人寿保险，以防意外。

integral ['intigrəl]　　　　*a.* 组成的，完整的，构成整体所需要的

integrity [in'tegriti]　　　　*n.* 诚实，正直，完整

【例句】They have always regarded man of integrity and fairness as a reliable friend.

【译文】他们一直认为诚实、正直的人是可信赖的朋友。

integrate ['intigreit]　　　　*vt.* 使结合，使一体化

【搭配】integrate...with... 把……与……相结合

integrate...into 使……并入

【例句】Many suggestions are need to integrate the plan.

【译文】需要许多建议使计划更加完整。

promote [prə'məut]　　　　*vt.* 提升，晋升；促进，增进，助长

【例句】They have greatly promoted American culture, and improved the living standards of the whole American people.

【译文】他们极大促进了美国文化的发展，提高了所有
美国人的生活水平。

proof [pruːf]   *n.* 证据，证明

property ['prɒpəti]   *n.* 财产，所/物；性质，特性
【搭配】movable/personal property 动产
       real property 不动产

proportion [prə'pɔːʃən]   *n.* 部分，份额；
                                 比例，比重；均衡，相称
【搭配】in proportion to 与······成比例
       out of proportion to 与······不成比例
【例句】Gradually raise the proportion of the tertiary
industry in the national economy.
【译文】逐步提高第三产业在国民经济中的比重。

proposal [prə'pəʊzəl]   *n.* 提议，建议；求婚
【导学】在 proposal 后的同位语从句和表语从句中，
谓语用虚拟语气。
【导学】辨析 proposal, suggest：proposal 意为"提
议，忠告"，指正式或通过一定程序或途径而
提出的建议；suggest 意为"建议"，指所提
建议不一定正确，仅供对方参考。

propose [prə'pəuz]　　　　　　*vt*. 提议，建议；求婚

【搭配】propose doing 建议做某事；propose to do 打算做某事；propose to sb. 向某人求婚

【导学】propose 的宾语从句中谓语用虚拟语气。

prostate ['prɔsteit]　　　　　　*n*. 前列腺

psychiatrist [sai'kaiətrist] *n*. 精神病医师，精神病学家

【导学】psychic 通灵的人；psychiatry 精神病学；psycho 精神病患者；psychology 心理学；psychologist 心理学家人＝试图用精神分析治疗病人的人＝psychiatrist 精神病学家，精神病医师

【例题】"The material on immigrant health shocked me when we first reviewed it." says panel member Arthus M. Kleinman, a psychiatrist and anthropologist at Harvard Medical School in Boston.

【译文】"当我们第一次审阅移民健康的资料时，我感到十分震惊。"审阅委员会的成员亚瑟 M. 克莱曼说。他是波士顿哈佛医学院的精神病学家和人类学家。

psychological [ˌsaikə'lɔdʒikəl]　　*a*. 心理（上）的，心理学的

publicity [pʌbˈlisiti]　*n.* 众所周知，闻名；宣传，广告

【联想】publication *n.* 发表，公布，出版

publicize [ˈpʌblisaiz]　　　　　*v.* 宣扬；引人注意；
广为宣传；推销

purchase [ˈpəːtʃəs]　　　*n.* 购买；购买的东西　*vt.* 购买

quarter [ˈkwɔːtə]　　　　*n.* 四分之一；一刻钟；季度

qualify [ˈkwɔlifai]　　*vt.* 取得资格，使合格，使胜任

【搭配】qualify as 有条件成为

【联想】qualification *n.* 资格，条件，限制，限定

Day 14

Day 15

intellect [ˈintilekt]　　　　　*n*. 理智，智力；有才智的人

intellectual [intiˈlektʃuəl]　　　　　　*n*. 知识分子
　　　　　　a. 智力的；显示智力的，能发挥才智的

【例题】 More legislation is needed to protect the
_____ property rights of the patent.
A. integrative　　　B. intellectual
C. intelligent　　　D. intelligible　　　B

【译文】需要更多立法保护专利知识产权。

intelligent [inˈtelidʒənt]　　　　　*a*. 聪明的，理智的

【联想】 intelligence *n*. 智力；理解力；情报，消息，
报道

【例题】 He was _____ enough to understand my
questions from the gestures I made.
A. intelligent　　　B. efficient
C. proficient　　　D. diligent　　　A

【译文】他非常聪明，能根据我的手势明白我的问题。

intelligible [inˈtelidʒəbl]　　　　　*a*. 可以理解的，
易领悟的，清晰的

【联想】 名词 intelligence 智慧，智力，智商
intelligible = intellig + ible（able）需要智慧才能理解的；intelligent 智慧的，聪明的

【例题】 This report would be <u>intelligible</u> only to an expert in computing.

A. intelligent   B. comprehensive

C. competent   D. comprehensible   D

【译文】 只有计算机专家才能明白这个报道。

intend [in'tend]   *vt.* 想要，打算，企图

【搭配】 intend to do sth. 打算做某事
be intended as/for 原意要，意指……

intense [in'tens]   *a.* 强烈的，激烈的，热烈的

intensive [in'tensiv]   *a.* 加强的，密集的；精工细作的

【导学】 辨析 intense，intensive：intense 意为"激烈的，强烈的"，如 intense competition（激烈的竞争）；intensive 意为"集中的，加强的"，如 intensive reading（精读）。

【例题】 The patient's health failed to such an extent that he was put into _____ care.

A. tense   B. rigid

C. intensive   D. tight   C

【译文】 这名病人的病情恶化得相当严重，因此对他进行了重病特别护理。

intention [in'tenʃən]　　　　　　*n.* 意图，意向，目的

【例题】 She had clearly no _____ of doing any
work, although she was very well paid.
A. tendency　　　B. ambition
C. intention　　　D. willingness　　　C

【译文】 她明显不打算干任何工作，尽管她的工资待遇
很不错。

interdispline [ˌintə'displin]　　　　　*n.* 交叉学科

【联想】 interdisplinary *a.* 交叉学科的

interface ['intə(ː)feis]　　　　　　*n.* 界面，接口

interactive [ˌintər'æktiv]　 *a.* 相互作用的，相互影响的

internal [in'tənl]　 *a.* 内的，内部的；国内的，内政的

【例句】 He suffered internal injuries in the accident.
【译文】 他在这次事故中受了内伤。

interpret [in'təːprit]　　 *vt.* 解释；说明；口译；翻译

【联想】 interpretation *n.* 解释，阐明
【导学】 辨析 translate，interpret：translate 指口头或
笔头翻译；interpret 仅指口头翻译。
【例句】 I interpret his answer as a refusal.
【译文】 我把他的回答理解为拒绝。

interrupt [ˌintəˈrʌpt]　　*vt.* 打断，打扰；断绝，中断

【导学】辨析 bankrupt, corrupt, interrupt：bankrupt
　　　　意为"破产的"；corrupt 意为"贪污的"；
　　　　interrupt 意为"中断，打断"。

interval [ˈintəvəl]　　　　　　　*n.* 间隔，间歇

【搭配】at intervals 有时，不时，时时；at an interval
　　　　of 间隔/间距（多长时间/多远）

intimate [ˈintimit]　　　　　　*a.* 亲密的，密切的

invade [inˈveid]　　　　*vt.* 侵入，侵略，侵害

【联想】invasion *n.* 侵入，侵略
【例句】She got annoyed when her colleague invaded
　　　　her privacy.
【译文】当同事侵犯她的隐私时，她很生气。

invalid [inˈvælid]　　*a.*（指法律上）无效的，作废的；
无可靠根据的，站不住脚的 *n.* (the) 病弱者，残疾者

【例句】Your license has been invalid.
【译文】你的执照已经作废了。

investigate [inˈvestigeit]　　　　*v.* 调查，调研

【搭配】investigate（into）sth. 对某事进行调查

irradiate [iˈreidieit]　　　　　　v. 照耀，辐射，(使)灿烂，(使)明亮

【例题】He rapidly became _____ with his own power in the team.

A. irrigated　　　B. irradiated

C. irritated　　　D. initial　　　B

【译文】他的能力让他很快在团队中脱颖而出。

irrational [iˈræʃnl]　　　　　a. 不合理的；不合逻辑的；没有道理的

【例句】She has an irrational dread of hospitals.

【译文】她莫名其妙地害怕医院。

ironic(al) [aiˈrɔnik(əl)]　　　a. 讽刺的，冷嘲的

irony [ˈairəni]　　　　　　n. 反话，讽刺

【例句】The irony of the historian's craft is that its practitioners always know that their efforts are but contributions to an unending process.

【译文】对历史学家技艺具有讽刺意味的是，参与实践者总是明白，他们的努力只是对一个无穷的过程的小小奉献。

isolate [ˈaisəleit]　　　　　vt. 隔离，孤立

【联想】isolation n. 隔离，孤立

【搭配】be isolated from 脱离，被隔离，被孤立

【例句】Several villages have been isolated by the floods.

【译文】洪水使好几座村庄与外界隔绝了。

obituary [ə'bitʃuəri]   *n.* 讣告 *a.* 死亡的，讣告的

obligation [ˌɔbli'geiʃən]   *n.* 义务；职责；责任

【搭配】be under no/an obligation（to do sth.）（没）有义务（做某事）

【例题】Parents have a legal _____ to ensure that their children are provided with efficient education suitable to their age.

A. impulse   B. influence

C. obligation   D. sympathy   C

【译文】父母在法律上有义务确保他们的孩子可以获得适合他们年龄的有效教育。

observe [əb'zə:v]   *vt.* 观察，注意到，看到；遵守，奉行；说，评论

【联想】observer *n.* 观察员

observation *n.* 观察，监视，评论，意见

【搭配】observe on/upon 评论

【例句】The scientist continues to experiment and

187

observe until the theories are proved.

【译文】这个科学家继续做实验并进行观察，直到这些理论被证明。

obstacle [ˈɔbstəkl]   *n.* 障碍

【例句】Materialism and individualism in American society are the biggest obstacles.

【译文】唯物主义和个人主义是美国社会最大的障碍。

obtain [əbˈtein]   *vt.* 获得，得到

occasion [əˈkeiʒən]   *n.* 场合；大事，节日；时机，机会

【搭配】on occasion 有时，偶尔
on the occasion of... 在……的时候

【联想】occasional *a.* 偶然的，不时的

occupation [ˌɔkjuˈpeiʃən]   *n.* 占领，职业

【联想】occupational *a.* 职业的

occupy [ˈɔkjupai]   *vt.* 占，占领，占据；
使忙碌，使从事

【搭配】occupy oneself in doing sth. /with sth. 忙着（做某事）；忙（于某事）；be occupied with/in 忙于

【例句】You were signaled forward to occupy the seat

opposite him.

【译文】有人暗示你向前去占他对面的座位。

operational [ˌɔpəˈreiʃnl]　　　*a.* 操作的，运作的

operator [ˈɔpəreitə]　　*n.* 操作人员；（电话）接线员

orphan [ˈɔːfən]　　　　　*n.* 孤儿 *a.* 无父母的

opponent [əˈpəunənt]　　　　　　*n.* 对手，敌手

【例题】We cannot look down upon our <u>opponent</u>, who is an experienced swimmer.
　　　A. player　　　　B. competitor
　　　C. referee　　　　D. partner　　　　B

【译文】我们不能轻视我们的对手，他是一名有经验的游泳选手。

opportunity [ˌɔpəˈtjuːniti]　　　　　*n.* 机会

【例句】About 60 percent of American adults nap when given the opportunity.

【译文】大约60%的美国成年人在有机会的时候会小睡一下。

oppose [əˈpəuz]　　　　　　　*vt.* 反对，反抗

【搭配】be opposed to sth. /doing sth. 反对

【例句】But they won't think this way; they will

oppose us stubbornly.

【译文】可是，他们不会这样想，他们要坚决反对我们。

optical [ˈɔptikəl]　　*a.* 光学的，光的；视觉的，视力的

oral [ˈɔːrəl]　　　　　　　　　*a.* 口头的，口的

【例句】This drug is available for both oral and parenteral administration.

【译文】本药可供口服或注射用。

organ [ˈɔːgən]　　　　　　　*n.* 器官；机构；风琴

【联想】organism *n.* 组织，机体

【例句】The FBI is an organ of the Justice Department.

【译文】联邦调查局是司法部的一个机构。

organic [ɔːˈgænik]　　　　　*a.* 有机体的，器官的

【搭配】organic food 有机食物

organize [ˈɔːgənaiz]　　　　　　*vt.* 组织，组编

【联想】organization *n.* 组织，体制；团体，机构

origin [ˈɔridʒin]　　　*n.* 起源，由来；出身，血统

【导学】辨析 origin，root，source：origin 指事物的起源或者开端，着重于其发生的最早的时间或最初的地点，常表示某种历史文化现象、风俗习惯的起源，也可指人的门第或血统；

root 常译为"根源，起因"，强调导致某事物最终出现的最根本的、最重要的原因，由此所产生的现象或事物常成为一种外观的产物；source 指河流或泉水的发源地，也是非物质的或无形的东西的出处或起源，常指情况或信息的来源、出处。

original [əˈridʒənəl]   *a*. 最初的，原始的，原文的；新颖的，有独创性的

【例句】 Internet was originally designed to promote education.

【译文】 互联网最初是为普及教育而设计的。

originate [əˈridʒineit]   *vt*. 引起，发明，发起，创办
    vi. 起源，发生

【搭配】 originate from/in/with 产生于

outbreak [ˈautbreik]   *n*. (战争、情感、火山等的)爆发；(疾病、虫害等的) 突然发生

【例句】 During the acute phase of the outbreak, it is necessary to keep suspects at special risk under observation.

【译文】 在爆发的急剧阶段，必须将面临特殊威胁的疑似病例置于监视之下。

overall [ˈəuvərɔːl]   *a.* 全面的，综合的

【例题】The _____ goal of the book is to help bridge the gap between research and teaching, particularly between researchers and teachers.

A. overall   B. intensive

C. joint   D. concise   A

【译文】这本书的总体目标是要帮助建立研究与教学之间的桥梁，尤其是要加强研究人员与老师之间的沟通。

Day *16*

label [ˈleibl]　*n.* 标签，标记 *v.* 贴标签，把……称为

【例句】 Is that label accurate? Is it intolerant to challenge another's opinion? It depends on what definition of opinion you have in mind.

【译文】 那个商标准确吗？去挑战他人的观点是否是偏执的呢？它完全取决于你心里对意见的定义。

【例题】 By the end of 1994，558 kinds of products had been _____ green food.
A. named　　　　B. restricted
C. classified　　D. labeled　　　　D

【译文】 到 1994 年年末，已经有 558 种产品被列为绿色食品。

laboratory [ləˈbɔrətəri]　　　　*n.* 实验室，研究室

largely [ˈlɑ:dʒli]　　　*ad.* 大部分，基本上；大规模地

laser [ˈleizə]　　　　　　　*n.* 激光

launch [lɔ:ntʃ]　　　*vt.* 发射；下水；开始，发起
　　　　　　　　　　　　n. 发射；下水

【搭配】launch an attack on/against 对……发动进攻

lawsuit ['lɔːsjuːt]   *n*. 诉讼

layer ['leiə]   *n*. 层

layoff ['leiɔːf]   *n*. (尤指临时) 解雇

layout ['leiaut]   *n*. 布局，安排，设计

leader ['liːdə]   *n*. 领袖，领导者

leadership ['liːdəʃip]   *n*. 领导

【搭配】under the leadership of 在……的领导下

leading ['liːdiŋ]   *a*. 指导的，领导的；
领先的；第……位的，最主要的

learned ['ləːnid]   *a*. 有学问的，博学的

legacy ['legəsi] *n*. 遗产；遗赠财物；遗留；后遗症

【例句】Future generations will be left with a legacy
of pollution and destruction.

【译文】留给子孙后代的将是环境的污染与破坏。

legal ['liːgl]   *a*. 合法的；法律的；
与法律有关的；法律允许的；法律要求的

legislation [ˌledʒis'leiʃən] *n.* 立法，法律的制定/通过

legislative ['ledʒisleitiv] *a.* 立法的，立法机关的
  n. 立法机关

legislator ['ledʒisleitə] *n.* 立法者

lethal ['liːθəl] *a.* 致命的，毁灭性的，有效的
  n. 基因异常，致死基因

【例题】 It has been proved that the chemical is <u>lethal</u> to rats but safe for cattle.
  A. fatal B. reactive
  C. unique D. vital A

【译文】 经证实，这种化学药品对于鼠类是致命的，但对家禽无害。

leukemia [luː'kiːmiə] *n.* 白血病

liable ['laiəbl] *a.* 有……倾向性，易于；有偿付责任的

【搭配】 be liable to 易于；be liable for 对……有责任

【例句】 A child can be born weak or liable to serious illness as a result of radiation.

【译文】 因为辐射，孩子刚刚出生就可能很虚弱或者易于罹患严重的疾病。

liability [ˌlaiə'biliti] *n.* 责任，义务；
  (*pl.*) 债务，负债

【搭配】liability for 对······有责任

liability to do 有责任做

【例句】A few common misconceptions：Beauty is only skin-deep. One's physical assets and liabilities don't count all that much in a managerial career.

【译文】有一些普遍的错误看法：美丽只是表面的。在管理职业生涯中，一个人外表的美丑并不意味着全部。

limitation [ˌlimiˈteiʃən]　　　　*n.* 缺陷，限额，限制

【例题】With all its advantages, the computer is by no means without its _____.

A. boundaries　　B. restraints

C. confinements　D. limitations　　D

【译文】尽管计算机有很多优点，但它也绝不是没有缺陷的。

limited [ˈlimitid]　　　　*a.* 被限定的，有限的

link [liŋk]　　　　*v.* 连接，联系 *n.* 环，链环；联系

liquid [ˈlikwid]　　　　*n.* 液体
a. 液体的，液态的；流动的；可兑换成现金的

【联想】solid *n.* 固体；gas *n.* 气体

liquor ['likə]　　　　　　　　　　　　　　*n*. 酒

literary ['litərəri] *a*. 文学的；精通文学的，从事写作的
【联想】literal *a*. 字面的，正确的，乏味的
　　　　literate *a*. 有文化的，识字的

literature ['litəritʃə]　　　　*n*. 文学，文学作品；文献
【搭配】contemporary literature 当代文学
　　　　light literature 通俗文学

loan [ləun]　　　　　　　*n*. 贷款 *v*. /*n*. 借出
【搭配】on loan 暂借的（地）

lubricate ['lu:brikeit]　　　　　*vt*. 润滑，加润滑油
【联想】lubrication *n*. 润滑；lubricator *n*. 润滑者
【例句】You should lubricate the wheels of your bicycle
　　　　once a month.
【译文】你应该每个月给自行车轮子加一次润滑油。

local ['ləukəl]　　　　　*a*. 地方的，当地的；局部的

locate [ləu'keit]　　*vt*. 找出，查出；设置在，位于
　　　　　　　　　　　　　　　　vi. 定居下来
【搭配】be located in/by/on 坐落于，位于
【例句】Early settlers located where there was water.
【译文】早期的移民者在有水的地方定居下来。

location [ləuˈkeiʃən]   *n.* 位置，地点；定位，测量

loyal [ˈlɔiəl]   *a.* 忠诚的，忠贞的

loyalty [ˈlɔiəlti]   *n.* 忠诚，忠心

【例句】 As a demanding boss, he expected total loyalty and dedication from his employees.

【译文】 他是个苛刻的老板，要求手下的人对他忠心耿耿、鞠躬尽瘁。

nasty [ˈnæsti]   *a.* 极令人不快的；很脏的；危险的

【导学】 和该词意思相反的是 pleasant（愉快的，可爱的）。

【例句】 Since the dawn of human ingenuity, people have devised ever more cunning tools to cope with work that is dangerous, boring, burdensome, or just plain nasty.

【译文】 自从人类灵智开发以来，就一直在设计越来越精巧的工具，去应付那些危险、枯燥、繁重或实在不堪忍受的各种劳动。

nausea [ˈnɔːziə]   *n.* 恶心，作呕，反胃

nearby [ˈniəbai]   *a. /ad.* 附近 *prep.* 在……附近

【导学】 nearby 既可以做前置定语，也可以做后置定语。辨析 nearby, near：nearby 指空间，不

指时间；near 可指时间和空间。

necessarily [nesi'serili]   *ad.* 必然，必定；当然

【搭配】not necessarily 未必（表部分否定）

necessity [ni'sesiti]   *n.* 必要性，必然性；必需品

【搭配】of necessity 无法避免地，必定

【导学】necessity 所接的表语从句或同位语从句的
        谓语常用"（should）＋动词原形"，表虚
        拟语气。

【例句】Is it a logical necessity that the cost of living
        will go up if wages go up?

【译文】如果工资提高生活费用就要上涨，这是逻辑的
        必然吗?

negative ['negətiv]   *a.* 否定的，消极的，反面的；
                              负的，阴性的

neglect [ni'glekt]   *vt.* 忽视，忽略；疏忽

【例句】The plan was negatived by the committee.

【译文】该计划被委员会否决了。

negotiate [ni'gəuʃieit]   *v.* 谈判，交涉，商议

【搭配】negotiate with sb. about/over/on/for sth. 与
        某人谈判某事

negotiable [ni'gəuʃiəbl]　　　　　*a*. 可谈判的，
可协商的，可通行的

neighbo(u)rhood ['neibəhud]　*n*. 邻近，附近，周围
【搭配】in the neighborhood of 在……附近，大约

neural ['njuərəl]　　　　　　*a*. 神经的，神经系统的

neutral ['njuːtrəl]　　　　　　*a*. 中立的，中性的
【例句】She is neutral in this argument. She does not care who wins.
【译文】在这场辩论中她保持中立，不在乎谁赢谁输。

normally ['nɔːməli]　　　　　　*ad*. 一般；通常
【例题】If your lively pets become passive，they might be ill _____ .
A. traditionally　　B. rarely
C. normally　　　　D. continually　　　C
【译文】如果你活泼好动的宠物变得怠惰，通常可能是它们病了。

normalize ['nɔːməlaiz]　　　　　*vt*. 使正常化，
使标准化，使规格化

notwithstanding [ˌnɔtwiθ'stændiŋ] *prep*. 虽然，尽管
ad. 尽管，还是 *conj*. 虽然，尽管

nuclear ['nu:kliə]   *a*. 原子核的；核的，核心的

【例句】Some scientists favor pushing asteroids off
course with nuclear weapons.

【译文】一些科学家更倾向于用核武器将行星从它们的
轨道推出去。

nutrition [nju:'triʃən]   *n*. 营养，营养学

【联想】nutritional *a*. 营养的

Day 17

machinery [mə'ʃiːnəri]   *n.* 机器；机关，结构

【导学】machine 是可数名词，表示机器；machinery
是不可数名词，表示机器的总称。

magic ['mædʒik]   *n.* 魔法，巫术；戏法

magnet ['mægnit]   *n.* 磁铁，磁石，磁体

magnetic [mæg'netik]   *a.* 磁的，有吸引力的

【例题】In order to be a successful diplomat you must
be enthusiastic and <u>magnetic</u>.

    A. arrogant   B. industrious

    C. zealous   D. attractive   D

【译文】想要成为一名成功的外交官，你必须热情且有
魅力。

magnetism ['mægnitizəm]   *n.* 磁，磁力，磁学

magnitude ['mægnitjuːd]   *n.* 巨大，重大；大小，数量

【联想】magnify *v.* 使……变大

【例题】The destruction an earthquake causes depends
on its _____ and duration, or the amount

of shaking that occurs.

A. altitude   B. magnitude

C. multitude   D. aptitude   B

【译文】地震造成的破坏程度由震级和持续的时间，或者震动发生的次数决定。

maintain [men'tein]   *vt.* 维持；赡养；维修

【例句】The leaders of the two countries are planning their summit meeting to maintain and develop good ties.

【译文】为保持并发展友好关系，两国的领导正在策划一场峰会。

maintenance ['meintinəns]   *n.* 维持，保持；维修

mainstream ['meinstri:m]   *n.* 主流

male [meil]   *a.* 男的，雄的 *n.* 男子

【联想】female *a.* 女的，雌性的

malpractice ['mæl'præktis]   *n.* 玩忽职守

management ['mænidʒmənt] *n.* 管理；经营，处理

mankind [mæn'kaind]   *n.* 人类

manifest ['mænifest]   *a.* 明显的，显然的，明了的
            vt. 明显，表明，证明；使显现，使显露

【例句】 The fact of first-rate importance is the predominant role that custom plays in experience and in belief and the very great varieties it may manifest.

【译文】 头等重要的事实就是风俗在信念和经验中所起的重要作用以及它所表现的众多变化形态。

manner ['mænə]　　　　　*n.* 方式；态度；礼貌

【搭配】 all manner of 各种各样的，形形色色的；in a manner of speaking 在某种意义上

【例句】 Manners on the roads are becoming horrible.

【译文】 大街上的行为正变得越来越可怕了。

manual ['mænjuəl]　　*a.* 用手的，手工的；体力的
　　　　　　　　　　　　　　　n. 手册

【例题】 The ship's generator broke down, and the pumps had to be operated _____ instead of mechanically.

　　　　 A. manually　　　 B. artificially

　　　　 C. automatically　 D. synthetically　　 A

【译文】 这艘船的发电机坏了，抽水机不能再机械运作了，必须由手工来操作。

manufacture [ˌmænju'fæktʃə]　　　　*vt.* 制造，加工
　　　　　　　　　　　　　　　　　　　n. 制造（业）；产品

manufacturer [ˌmænjuˈfæktʃərə]　　　　*n*. 制造者，制造商；制造厂

manipulate [məˈnipjuleit]　　*vt*. 操纵，利用，操作，巧妙地处理

【例句】 In this exercise, we'll look at how we can manipulate the columns and rows in a table.

【译文】 在此练习中，我们将了解如何处理表中的列和行。

margin [ˈmɑːdʒin]　　　　*n*. 页边空余；边缘；利润

【联想】 marginal *a*. 边缘的

【例题】 You shouldn't have written in the _____ since the book belongs to the library.

  A. interval B. border

  C. margin D. edge C

【译文】 既然这本书是属于图书馆的，你就不应该在页边空白处写字。

marine [məˈriːn]　　　　*a*. 海的，海产的，航海的，船舶的，海运的

marvellous [ˈmɑːviləs]　　　　*a*. 奇迹般的，惊人的，了不起的

【导学】 辨析 marvellous, wonderful：marvellous 形

容非凡得令人难以置信的东西；wonderful
指因未曾见过或不寻常而令人惊奇。

mature [mə'tjuə]　　　　　*a.* 成熟的，考虑周到的
　　　　　　　　　　　　　　v. (使)成熟，长成

【联想】immature *a.* 不成熟的；maturity *n.* 成熟

【导学】辨析 mature，ripe：mature 用于人时，指生
　　　　理和智力发展到了成年，用于物时，指机能
　　　　发展到可以开花结果，还可指想法、意图等
　　　　"经过深思熟虑的"；ripe 用于物时，指植物
　　　　的果实完全成熟，可以食用，也可指时机
　　　　"成熟的，适宜的"。

【例句】Boys mature more slowly than girls both
　　　　physically and psychologically.

【译文】无论在生理上或心理上，男孩都比女孩成熟
　　　　得晚。

maximum ['mæksiməm]　　　　*n.* 最大量，最高值
　　　　　　　　　　　　　　　a. 最大的，最高的

【联想】minimum *n./a.* 最小(量)

【导学】maximum 的复数形式为 maxima 或 maximums。

【例句】The level of formaldehyde (甲醛) gas in her
　　　　kitchen was twice the maximum allowed by
　　　　federal standard for chemical workers.

【译文】在她家厨房，甲醛的浓度是联邦政府为化工厂

的工人规定的最高标准的两倍。

means [miːnz]　　　　　　　　*n*. 方法，手段，工具

【搭配】by all means 当然；by any means 无论如何；
by no means 决不；by means of 用，凭借

【联想】in any case, at any cost, one way or the
other 无论如何；under no circumstances，in
no respect，in no sense，in no way，on no
account，at no time 绝不

【例题】Though _____ rich, he was better off than
at any other period in his life.
A. by any means　　B. by some means
C. by all means　　D. by no means　　D

【译文】尽管生活并不富裕，但他过得比以往任何时候
都好。

meantime [ˈmiːnˈtaim]　　　　*n*. 其时，在此期间
　　　　　　　　　　　　　　　　ad. 同时，当时

measurement [ˈmeʒəmənt]　　*n*. 测量，度量；
　　　　　　　　　　　　　　　　尺寸，大小

【联想】measure *vt*. 测量

mechanic [miˈkænik]　　　　*n*. 技工，机械工人

mechanical [miˈkænikl]　　　*a*. 机械的；机械学的，
　　　　　　　　　　　　　　　　力学的；机械似的，呆板的

mechanism ['mekənizəm] *n.* 机械装置；机构，结构
n. 奖章，勋章，纪念章

medium ['mi:djəm] *n.* 中间，适中；(*pl.* media)
媒体；媒介，媒介物；传导体 *a.* 中等的，适中的

【导学】medium 的复数形式为 media。类似的词还有 datum—data。但 应 注 意 premium— premiums；gymnasium—gymnasiums。

【例句】He is medium height.

【译文】他是中等身材。

mediate ['mi:diit] *v.* 仲裁，调停

medical ['medikl] *a.* 医学的；医疗的；伤病的；疾病的；内科的 *n.* 体格检查

【例句】Therapists cannot prescribe drugs as they are not necessarily medically qualified.

【译文】由于治疗师不一定具有行医资格，所以他们不可以开处方。

medication [ˌmedi'keiʃn] *n.* 药物

mental ['mentl] *a.* 思想的；精神的；思考的；智力的；精神病治疗的；精神健康的；疯狂的；发疯的
n. 精神病；精神病患者

mentality [men'tæləti]　　　　　*n*. 心态，思想方式

【例句】I cann't understand their mentality.

【译文】我理解不了他们的心态。

metabolism [me'tæbəlizəm]　　　　*n*. 新陈代谢

【例题】Diabetes upsets the _____ of sugar, fat and protein.

　　　　A. metastasis　　B. metabolism

　　　　C. malaise　　　D. maintenance　　　B

【译文】糖尿病扰乱了糖、脂肪和蛋白质的代谢。

methane ['mi:θein]　　　　　　*n*. 甲烷，沼气

migrate [mai'greit]　　　*v*. 迁移，迁居；定期移栖

【联想】migrant *n*. 移居者；候鸟

【例句】We find that some birds migrate twice a year between hot and cold countries.

【译文】我们发现，有些鸟每年在热带与寒带国家之间迁徙两次。

millimeter ['milimi:tə(r)]　　　　　*n*. 毫米

miniature ['minjətʃə]　　　　　*n*. 缩图，缩影

　　　　　　　　　　　　　　　a. 微型的，缩小的

【例句】The toy maker produces a miniature copy of the space station，exactly in every detail.

【译文】 这个玩具制造商制造了一种每个细节都很逼真的空间站缩微模型。

minimal ['miniməl]　　　　　*a.* 最小的，最小限度的

minimum ['miniməm]　　　　*n.* 最小量，最低限度
　　　　　　　　　　　　　　　a. 最小的，最低的

【例句】 He said China would reduce losses incurred by SARS to the minimum.

【译文】 他说中国会把 SARS 引起的损失降到最小程度。

mislead [mis'li:d]　　　　*vt.* 使误入歧途；
　　　　　　　　　　　　　　　把……带错路；使误解

missile ['misail]　　　　　*n.* 发射物；导弹

missing ['misiŋ]　　　　　*a.* 失去的，失踪的

【例题】 John complained to the bookseller that there were several pages _____ in the dictionary he bought.
　　　　A. missing　　　　B. losing
　　　　C. dropping　　　　D. leaking　　　　A

【译文】 约翰向书商抱怨说，他买的字典少了几页。

mission ['miʃən]　　　　　*n.* 使命，任务

【搭配】 on a...mission 负有……使命

misunderstand [ˈmisʌndəˈstænd] *vt.* 误解，误会，曲解

mitigage [ˈmitigeit]   *vt.* 减轻；缓和
【例句】It would help mitigate your discomfort.
【译文】这会帮你缓解不适。

moderate [ˈmɔdərit]   *a.* 中等的，适度的；温和的，
                                         稳健的

moral [ˈmɔrəl]   *a.* 道德的，道义的，有道德的
                                n. 寓意，教育意义
【联想】morality *n.* 道德
【例句】As regards the development of moral stand-
        ards in the growing child, consistency is very
        important in parental teaching.
【译文】对于在成长中的孩子的道德水平的发展，一致
        性是非常重要的。

motivate [ˈmɔutiveit] *vt.* 作为……的动机，促动；激励
【例句】Examinations do not motivate a student to
        seek more knowledge.
【译文】考试不能促使学生去追求更多的知识。

motive [ˈmɔutiv] *n.* 动机，目的 *a.* 发动的，运动的

mutation [mju:ˈteiʃn] *n.* 突变；（生物种的）变异；
                             （形式或结构的）转变；改变

【例句】The virus mutates in the carrier's body.

【译文】病毒在在载体中发生了变异。

mutant [ˈmjuːtənt]　　　　　　　　*a.* 变异的，突变的

【例句】The experts said the new vaccine can produce neutralizing antibodies for mutant COVID-19 strains found in Brazil.

【译文】专家们说，这种新疫苗可以产生针对巴西发现的 COVID-19 突变株的中和抗体。

mutual [ˈmjuːtjuəl]　　　　　　　　*a.* 相互的；共同的

【例句】He had taken the all-important first step to establish mutual trust.

【译文】为了建立相互信任关系，他迈出了最重要的第一步。

Day 18

vacant ['veikənt] *a.* 空的；（职位）空缺的；茫然的

【联想】vacancy *n.* 空缺

【例句】Are there any rooms vacant in this hotel?

【译文】这家旅馆有空房吗？

vaccine ['væksiːn] *a.* 疫苗的，牛痘的 *n.* 疫苗

【联想】vaccinate *v.*（给……）接种（疫苗）；（给……）打预防针

【例题】Figures like these bring home the devastating impact of AIDS and the urgent need for a cheap, effective vaccine.

【译文】这样的数据让人们了解了艾滋病毁灭性影响，人们急需一种廉价有效的疫苗。

vacuum ['vækjuəm] *n.* 真空；真空吸尘器

【例句】Her death left a vacuum in his life.

【译文】她的去世给他的生活留下一片真空。

variable ['vɛəriəbl] *n.* 变量 *a.* 易变的；可变的，可调节的

variation [ˌvɛəriˈeiʃən] *n.* 变化，变动；变种，变异

vary ['veəri]　　　　　　　　　*vt.* 变化，改变

【搭配】vary with... 随……变化；vary from...to...
　　　　由……到……情况不同

【例题】The hopes, goals, fears and desires _____
　　　　widely between men and women, between
　　　　the rich and the poor.
　　　　A. alter　　　　　B. transfer
　　　　C. shift　　　　　D. vary　　　　　D

【译文】无论男女，无论贫富，每个人的希望、目标、
　　　　忧虑和愿望都大不相同。

vehicle ['viːikl]　　　　　　*n.* 车辆，交通工具

【例句】Cars and trucks are vehicles.

【译文】小汽车和大卡车都是交通工具。

venture ['ventʃə]　　　*n. /vi.* 冒险，拼，闯
　　　　　　　　　　v. 敢于，大胆表示 *n.* 冒险（事业）

【搭配】at a venture 胡乱地，随便地

【导学】辨析 venture，adventure，risk：venture 指冒
　　　　生命危险或经济风险；adventure 指使人心振
　　　　奋、寻求刺激性的冒险；risk 指不顾个人安
　　　　危、主动承担风险的事。

verify ['verifai]　　　　*vt.* 证实，证明；查清，核实

【例题】There are often discouraging predictions that

have not been _____ by actual events.

A. verified　　　　B. utilized

C. mobilized　　　D. modified　　A

【译文】经常会有未经事实证明的令人沮丧的预测。

veteran ['vetərən]　　　*n.* 老兵，老手 *a.* 老练的

via ['vaiə]　　　　　*prep.* 经，经由，通过

【例句】I went to Pittsburgh via Philadelphia.

【译文】我经过费城到匹兹堡。

vibrate [vai'breit]　　*v.* (使) 振动，(使) 摇摆

【联想】vibration *n.* 振动

【例句】The diaphragm vibrates, thus setting the air around it in motion.

【译文】膜片振动使得周围的空气也动荡起来。

violate ['vaiəleit]　　*vt.* 违犯，违背，违例

【联想】violation *n.* 违反

【搭配】violate the regulation/agreement 违反规定/协约

【例题】The actress _____ the terms of her contract and was prosecuted by the producer.

A. ignored　　　　B. ratified

C. drafted　　　　D. violated　　D

【译文】这位女演员违反了她合同的所有条款，因此被

制片人起诉了。

virtual ['vɜːtjuəl]   *a*. 虚的，虚拟的；实际上的

【联想】virtually *ad*. 实际上

virtue ['vɜːtjuː]   *n*. 美德；优点

【搭配】by/in virtue of 借助，经由

【例题】The manager spoke highly of such _____ as loyalty, courage and truthfulness shown by his employees.

A. virtues   B. features

C. properties   D. characteristics   A

【译文】经理高度评价员工所表现出的忠诚、勇气和诚实等美德。

virus ['vaiərəs]   *n*. 病毒

【例句】This is the pernicious virus of racism.

【译文】这是种族主义的毒害。

vision ['viʒən]   *n*. 视觉，视力；幻想，幻影；眼力，想象力；远见

【导学】辨析 vision, sight, view: vision 指人的视力或视野，引申为远见卓识、美妙景色等；sight 指事物在人视线中的客观映象，引申为奇观、风景名胜等；view 指视线、视野时，可与 sight 互换使用，但 view 可指运用视力

直接观察事物，也可指问题的角度、个人意见、美景等。

visual ['viʒuəl]   *a.* 视觉的

vital ['vaitl]   *a.* 极其重要的，致命的；生命的；有生机的

【搭配】be vital to 对……极其重要
【导学】It's vital that 从句谓语动词用原形表示虚拟形式。
【例句】The young people are the most active and vital force in society.
【译文】青年是社会中最活跃、最有生气的力量。

vitamin ['vaitəmin]   *n.* 维生素

voluntary ['vɔləntri]   *a.* 自愿的 *n.* 自愿者

【例句】There is a voluntary conveyance of property.
【译文】这是一桩自愿的财产转让。

volunteer [vɔlən'tiə(r)]   *n.* 志愿者，志愿兵

vulnerable ['vʌlnərəb(ə)l]   *a.* 易受攻击的，有弱点的；易受伤害的，脆弱的

【搭配】vulnerable to 易受伤害的，易受打击的（其中 to 为介词，后面需接名词或名词短语）

【例句】 Some researchers feel that certain people have nervous systems particularly vulnerable to hot, dry winds. They are what we call weather-sensitive people.

【译文】 一些研究人员认为，有些人的神经系统特别容易受到干燥的热风的影响，他们就是我们所说的对天气敏感的人。

wisdom ['wizdəm] *n.* 智慧，明智；名言，格言；古训

withdraw [wið'drɔː]   *vt.* 收回；撤回，提取
　　　　　　　　　　　　　vi. 撤退，退出

【联想】 withdrawal *n.* / *a.* 撤回（的）

【搭配】 withdraw...from... 将……从……撤回
　　　　 withdraw from 退出

【例句】 If after education he or she still shows no change, the Party branch shall persuade him or her to withdraw from the Party.

【译文】 经教育仍无转变的人，党支部应当劝其退党。

withstand [wið'stænd]   *vt.* 抵抗，经受住

【例句】 The new beach house on Sullivan's Island should be able to withstand a Category 3 hurricane with peak winds of 179 to 209 kilometers per hour.

【译文】 在沙利文岛的海边房屋应该能够抵挡 3 级飓

风，这种飓风的最高风速为每小时 179～209
公里。

worthless ['wəːθlis]　　　　*a*. 无价值的，无用的

worthwhile ['wəːð'(h)wail]　　　*a*. 值得（做）的

worthy ['wəːði]　*a*. 有价值的，可尊敬的；值……的，
　　　　　　　　　　　　　　　　足以……的

【搭配】 be worthy of... 值得……的
　　　　 be worthy to do... 值得去做……
【联想】 it is worthwhile to do sth. /sth. is worth
　　　　 doing 值得做某事
【导学】 sth. is worth（doing）（接名词或动名词）
　　　　 sth. is worthy to be done（接不定式）
　　　　 sth. is worthy of（接 of 短语）
　　　　 it is worthwhile to do sth.（接不定式做主语）
　　　　 sth. is deserving of（接 of 短语）

wreck [rek]　　　　　*n*. 失事，遇难；沉船，残骸
　　　　　　　　　　　vt.（船等）失事，遇难

【例句】 He escaped from the train wreck without
　　　　 injury.
【译文】 他在这次火车事故中没有受伤。

wrist [rist]　　　　　　　*n*. 腕，腕关节

【联想】 ankle *n*. 踝，踝关节；pulse *n*. 脉搏；palm
n. 手掌；finger *n*. 手指；toe *n*. 脚趾

X-ray ['eks'rei]   *n*. X 射线，X 光

yearly ['jə:li]   *a*. 每年的，一年一度的

yield [ji:ld]   *vt*. 生产，出产；让步，屈服
                            vi. 屈服，服从 *n*. 产量，收获量

【搭配】 yield to 向……让步
        increase the yield 增加产量

【联想】 submit *v*. 屈服；obey *v*. 服从；compromise
        v. 妥协；surrender *v*. 投降

【例句】 They were short of sticks to make frames for
        the climbing vines，without which the yield
        would be halved.

【译文】 他们缺少搭葡萄架的杆儿，没有它们葡萄产量
        就会减少一半。

zone [zəun]   *n*. 地带，区域

【例句】 Which time zone is your city located in?
【译文】 你们的城市位于哪个时区？

wealthy ['welθi]   *a*. 富裕的，富有的，富庶的

【例句】 He made his country wealthy and powerful.
【译文】 他使国家富强了。

whatsoever [wɔtsəu'evə(r)] = whatever

                               pron. 无论什么

whereas [(h)wɛər'æz]　*conj.* 鉴于；然而，但是；反之

widespread ['waidspred]

                               a. 普遍的，分布/散布广的

【例句】SARS is not a widespread disease.

【译文】SARS 并不是一个广泛传播的疾病。

附录一

医博英语真题词汇词频统计表

本词汇表为近十年真题试卷中词频在 30 以上的单词，使用的统计软件为 Wordcount。统计时同词根的派生词、合成词均独立计算，比如 she 和 she's 计算成两个词，分别统计词频。

单词	频率	单词	频率
the	4493	be	529
to	2260	on	467
of	2086	you	427
and	1411	have	424
in	1366	with	420
is	1182	what	404
that	850	as	400
for	669	from	385
it	568	can	371
are	550	not	315

单词	频率	单词	频率
more	309	than	183
by	306	has	182
their	304	people	178
but	303	how	175
at	299	there	164
they	292	no	155
he	285	had	149
about	270	if	148
we	263	most	148
or	251	were	147
this	245	so	145
was	232	all	144
will	227	new	144
an	226	who	141
do	212	when	138
passage	206	been	135
which	197	your	135
his	196	some	134
she	193	would	132
one	184	our	131

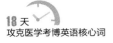

（续）

单词	频率	单词	频率
may	129	up	105
does	129	my	104
out	127	now	103
man	126	many	102
health	123	woman	101
two	121	well	101
just	117	according	100
her	117	work	99
could	117	says	98
research	116	study	98
it's	116	these	97
because	115	day	95
patient	113	them	94
should	112	cancer	93
time	112	children	93
other	110	need	90
take	110	much	85
medical	110	way	85
following	109	scientist	84
like	107	part	84

单词	频率	单词	频率
sleep	82	such	71
disease	81	author	71
year	81	help	70
only	80	medicine	70
use	79	even	70
between	78	think	70
get	78	three	70
over	78	too	69
why	76	care	69
good	76	did	69
its	76	researcher	68
doctor	76	problem	68
long	76	those	68
also	75	effect	68
first	73	don't	67
any	73	make	67
human	72	brain	66
world	72	change	66
me	72	very	66
into	71	better	65

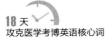

(续)

单词	频率	单词	频率
found	64	system	55
weight	64	genetic	54
science	63	last	54
question	62	patient	53
where	62	high	53
see	62	being	53
less	61	going	53
say	61	important	52
then	60	life	52
before	60	development	52
after	59	still	52
cell	58	test	52
know	58	different	51
based	57	likely	51
year	57	go	51
us	57	blood	51
best	57	mean	50
university	57	women	50
food	57	energy	50
right	56	problem	49

单词	频率	单词	频率
might	49	really	41
said	48	used	41
climate	48	made	41
same	48	pain	40
off	46	got	40
often	46	through	40
feel	45	drug	40
both	45	result	40
answer	44	talk	40
question	44	effect	40
little	44	animal	40
risk	44	scientific	40
liver	44	information	38
him	44	bad	38
during	43	body	38
own	43	find	38
American	43	while	38
probably	42	around	38
doctor	42	time	38
student	42	school	37

（续）

单词	频率	单词	频率
obesity	37	million	34
here	37	eye	34
already	37	become	34
lot	37	cause	34
anything	37	yes	34
number	37	human	34
country	37	exercise	34
Dr	37	must	34
case	37	come	34
physical	36	age	34
give	36	future	34
global	35	reason	34
treatment	35	paragraph	34
want	35	true	33
diabetes	35	percent	33
learn	35	heart	33
family	35	child	33
result	35	possible	33
among	35	disease	33
surgery	35	enough	33

单词	频率	单词	频率
difficult	32	education	31
taking	32	another	30
every	32	four	30
few	32	lab	30
each	32	drug	30
today	32	home	30
great	32	against	30
tell	32	usually	30
example	32	culture	30
parent	32	can't	30
job	31	what's	29
studies	31	lower	29
having	31	type	29
caffeine	31	day	29
back	31	birth	29
without	31	feeling	29
eat	31	computer	29
needs	31	down	29
several	31	place	29
however	31	heard	29

（续）

单词	频率	单词	频率
develop	28	exposure	27
current	28	changes	27
growing	28	HIV	27
known	28	water	27
under	28	almost	27
understand	28	able	27
impact	28	way	27
doing	28	loss	27
public	28	idea	26
past	28	hard	26
understanding	28	actually	26
next	28	sick	26
white	28	serious	26
early	28	five	26
put	28	sperm	26
effective	28	look	26
something	28	whether	26
thinking	27	yet	26
pill	27	social	26
reduce	27	week	26

单词	频率	单词	频率
young	26	ago	25
means	26	meat	24
old	26	model	24
healthy	26	green	24
thing	26	expected	24
clinical	25	others	24
infection	25	adult	24
men	25	insulin	24
cannot	25	virus	24
therapy	25	sleeping	24
history	25	hour	24
market	25	rate	24
live	25	never	24
biological	25	environment	24
low	25	obese	24
behavior	25	learning	24
second	25	seems	24
diet	25	always	24
stay	25	doesn't	24
experience	25	least	23

（续）

单词	频率	单词	频率
skill	23	month	22
emission	23	increase	22
fat	23	sometimes	22
man's	23	morning	22
makes	23	smoking	22
developed	23	finding	22
developing	23	dialogue	22
making	23	short	22
animal	23	hospital	22
neuron	23	knowledge	22
far	23	using	22
end	23	value	22
report	23	comprehension	22
given	23	program	22
environmental	23	term	22
since	22	country	21
treated	22	begin	21
taken	22	big	21
evidence	22	side	21
growth	22	conversation	21

单词	频率	单词	频率
reported	21	half	20
mother	21	cost	20
poor	21	once	20
start	21	college	20
united	21	week	20
flu	21	building	20
person	21	try	20
stress	21	small	20
suggest	21	test	20
further	21	higher	20
highly	21	reading	20
prevent	21	phone	20
level	21	eating	20
general	21	matter	20
thing	21	kid	20
factor	21	describe	20
technology	21	sure	20
state	21	provide	20
left	21	mind	20
trying	20	John	20

（续）

单词	频率	单词	频率
training	20	rather	19
show	20	inferred	19
issue	20	let's	19
thought	20	levels	19
available	20	safe	19
greater	20	ten	19
product	19	particular	19
senior	19	suggests	19
keep	19	difference	19
company	19	avoid	19
art	19	started	19
real	19	working	19
condition	19	beginning	19
activity	19	diagnosis	19
group	19	negative	19
mental	19	lack	19
fact	19	woman's	19
ability	19	recent	19
set	19	common	19
although	19	quality	19

单词	频率	单词	频率
haven't	19	pay	18
face	19	rat	18
hour	19	case	18
called	19	affect	18
wonder	19	within	18
form	19	community	18
donor	18	coffee	18
illness	18	stop	18
issue	18	mobile	18
immune	18	bit	18
control	18	data	18
open	18	healthcare	18
hormone	18	six	18
roof	18	away	18
kind	18	view	18
whole	18	fever	18
room	18	team	18
drink	18	ask	18
later	18	function	18
increased	18	simply	18

（续）

单词	频率	单词	频率
safety	18	product	17
practice	18	done	17
longer	18	seem	17
game	17	radiation	17
published	17	family	17
potential	17	structure	17
soon	17	nothing	17
lung	17	average	17
worry	17	role	17
night	17	sense	17
eye	17	American	17
news	17	weather	17
sample	17	clear	17
depression	17	shows	16
com	17	nature	16
until	17	success	16
project	17	machine	16
relationship	17	benefit	16
getting	17	carbon	16
turn	17	scientist	16

单词	频率	单词	频率
clinic	16	subject	16
penicillin	16	led	16
death	16	non	16
title	16	giving	16
gene	16	antibiotic	16
examination	16	Chinese	15
dangerous	16	whose	15
caused	16	offer	15
treat	16	word	15
vaccine	16	drink	15
pressure	16	lead	15
though	16	action	15
easy	16	citizen	15
cell	16	middle	15
perhaps	16	quite	15
looking	16	particularly	15
population	16	response	15
air	16	build	15
again	16	gene	15
listening	16	lives	15

（续）

单词	频率	单词	频率
living	15	hope	15
government	15	robot	15
play	15	European	15
isn't	15	cough	15
read	15	mentioned	15
severe	15	claims	15
service	15	attention	15
vision	15	hear	15
month	15	mainly	15
olds	15	business	14
began	15	wrong	14
necessary	15	course	14
biology	15	especially	14
large	15	listen	14
cognitive	15	class	14
alone	15	self	14
believe	15	term	14
infected	15	company	14
consumer	15	produce	14
tourism	15	German	14

单词	频率	单词	频率
international	14	creativity	14
portal	14	society	14
normal	14	advance	14
improve	14	physician	14
strong	14	caregiver	14
increasing	14	plan	14
children's	14	earlier	14
member	14	word	14
along	14	takes	14
baby	14	ones	14
fast	14	eight	14
theory	14	pill	14
beef	14	stomach	14
works	14	supposed	14
hand	14	management	14
area	14	recently	14
worker	14	technology	14
phones	14	job	14
else	14	laboratory	14
reality	14	money	14

（续）

单词	频率	单词	频率
didn't	14	hungry	13
journal	14	daughter	13
car	14	free	13
modern	14	finding	13
follow	14	comes	13
fear	13	specific	13
discovered	13	evolution	13
ear	13	summer	13
consumption	13	genome	13
due	13	showed	13
shown	13	critical	13
cold	13	coming	13
successful	13	specialist	13
specialist	13	antibody	13
similar	13	late	13
Smith	13	redux	13
effort	13	came	13
smaller	13	journal	13
stem	13	operation	13
emotional	13	involved	13

单词	频率	单词	频率
became	13	label	13
positive	13	major	13
physician	13	liver	13
amount	13	friend	12
address	13	childhood	12
bite	13	teaching	12
asked	13	ray	12
vaccination	13	designed	12
minute	13	feet	12
lose	13	art	12
call	13	doctor's	12
patient's	13	adult	12
treatment	13	she's	12
link	13	symptom	12
process	13	he's	12
move	13	condition	12
warming	13	African	12
bed	13	cancer	12
warning	13	rise	12
mice	13	wife	12

（续）

单词	频率	单词	频率
analysis	12	abuse	12
certain	12	difference	12
present	12	department	12
concerns	12	generalist	12
rule	12	let	12
approach	12	costs	12
UK	12	respond	12
themselves	12	combination	12
itself	12	brain	12
behind	12	stage	12
scale	12	decade	12
trouble	12	colleague	12
despite	12	hearing	12
thinks	12	coli	12
ever	12	born	12
period	12	lived	12
access	12	heat	12
China	12	danger	12
Vinci	12	natural	12
practice	12	including	12

单词	频率	单词	频率
violent	12	telehealth	11
remain	12	unique	11
together	12	technical	11
Chinatown	12	subject	11
helps	12	anti	11
personal	12	music	11
mechanism	12	antibiotic	11
improved	12	noise	11
chronic	12	COPD	11
prenatal	11	suffering	11
creative	11	California	11
twice	11	tendency	11
fen	11	lost	11
Henry	11	teach	11
Wainwright	11	significant	11
focus	11	heavy	11
main	11	contamination	11
dioxide	11	reason	11
sleepwalking	11	died	11
appointment	11	bring	11

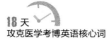
（续）

单词	频率	单词	频率
benefit	11	importance	11
happen	11	resistance	11
thanks	11	pattern	11
local	11	cloze	11
ulcer	11	you've	11
vocabulary	11	above	11
milk	11	infection	11
vegetative	11	author's	11
medication	11	aware	11
measure	11	injury	11
grant	11	species	11
either	11	demand	11
gave	11	English	11
party	11	deal	11
damage	11	goes	11
point	11	institute	11
chemistry	11	indeed	11
chemical	11	outbreak	11
game	11	traditional	11
check	11	planet	11

单词	频率	单词	频率
cut	11	challenge	11
group	11	throughout	11
shape	11	related	10
online	11	walk	10
full	11	suggested	10
conducted	11	sensitive	10
extreme	11	saw	10
moment	11	system	10
car	11	crucial	10
talking	11	cure	10
smiles	11	susceptible	10
argues	11	maintain	10
failure	11	defect	10
faint	11	Freud	10
quickly	11	nearly	10
gain	11	surgical	10
changing	11	surgeon	10
phen	11	measure	10
greenhouse	11	name	10
order	11	assage	10
idea	11	bacteria	10
easily	11	Arctic	10

（续）

单词	频率	单词	频率
wait	10	Africa	10
seek	10	causes	10
tablet	10	agree	10
meal	10	red	10
national	10	AIDS	10
black	10	policy	10
psychologist	10	conference	10
bitten	10	everything	10
serve	10	influence	10
stock	10	spilled	10
they're	10	total	10
implies	10	spent	10
immigrant	10	indicate	10
economy	10	combined	10
economic	10	took	10
exposome	10	overweight	10
extra	10	instead	10
completely	10	huge	10
confirmed	10	stand	10
perspective	10	part	10
pig	10	sparrow	10
reduced	10	interest	10

单词	频率	单词	频率
parental	10	feedback	10
compared	10	finally	10
paint	10	building	10
investment	10	nice	10
insomnia	10	wealth	10
ant	10	brought	10
method	10	seemed	10
antiretroviral	10	break	10
student	10	home	10
Wednesday	10	popular	10
leukemia	10	hold	10
tend	10	Hitler	10
rate	10	temperature	10
ready	10	stroke	10

注：由于篇幅所限，无法罗列全文。

请根据封面指示获取词频统计表全文电子版。

附录二

高频基础词汇表

从附录一中的词频统计不难看出，在真题中高频出现的往往是我们在复习备考中容易忽视的初高中基础词汇。因此，我们将高中基础词汇（附常见搭配和用法总结）做成了电子版，如下所示：

a	*art*. 一（个）；每一（个）；（同类事物中的）任何一个
ability	*n*. 能力，智能；才能，才干
	拓展 able—unable 不能的
	ability—inability 无能
	enable—disable 使无能，使残废
able	*a*. 有能力的；能干的
	拓展 be able to do sth. 能做，会做
	have the ability to do sth. 有做……的能力
aboard	*ad*. & *prep*. 在船（车、飞行器）上，上船（车、飞行器）
about	*prep*. 关于，对于；在……周围，在……附近 *ad*. 在周围，附近；大约，差不多
	拓展 be about to（do）即将（不跟表示将来的时

间状语)

above	*prep*. 在……上面，超过 *a*. 上面的，上述的 *ad*. 在上面，以上
	拓展 above all 首先，尤其
abroad	*ad*. 国外，海外；传开
	拓展 at home and abroad 国内外
abstract	*n*. 摘要，梗概；抽象派艺术作品
	v. 做……的摘要；提取，抽取
	a. 抽象的，抽象派的
according to	*prep*.（表示依据）根据，按照
across	*ad*. / *prep*. 横越，横断 *prep*. 在……对面
act	*n*. 行为，动作；（一）幕；法令，条例
	v. 行动，举动；起作用；表演
	拓展 act on/upon 按……行动；对……起作用
	act as 担任，充当
action	*n*. 行动；作用
	拓展 out of action 失去作用；有故障
	take action 采取行动
active	*a*. 活动的，活跃的；积极的，主动的
activity	*n*. 活动；活力；行动
actor	*n*. 演员，男演员；行动者
actress	*n*. 女演员
add	*vt*. 加，加上；增加，增进；进一步说/写
	vi. 增添

附录二

拓展 add to 增加，添加，补充

add（up）to ＝ total（up）to 总计，等于；
意指

注：由于篇幅所限，无法罗列全文。
请根据封面指示获取基础词汇表全文电子版。